HALF

The Woman

I WAS

How I lost **70kg (154lbs) naturally**,
reclaimed my life …
and how you can too!

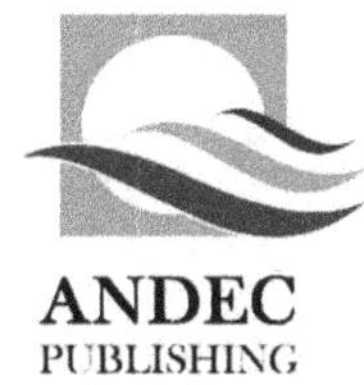

ANDEC
PUBLISHING

HALF

The Woman

I WAS

How I lost **70kg (154lbs) naturally**,
reclaimed my life …
and how you can too!

Sigrid de Castella

DISCLAIMER

This book is written as a source of information only. Neither the publisher nor the author are engaged
in rendering medical advice to the individual reader. The information contained in this book should by
no means be considered a substitute for advice by a qualified medical professional, who should always
be consulted before beginning and new diet, exercise or health program. Every effort has been made
to ensure the accuracy of the information in this book. The author and the publisher expressly disclaim
responsibility for any adverse effects arising from the use or application of the information contained herein.

For further information please contact:
www.HalfTheWomanIWas.com
Email: info@halfthewomaniwas.com

National Library of Australia
Cataloguing-in publication data

de Castella, Sigrid
Half The Woman I Was
How I lost 70kg (154lbs) naturally, reclaimed my life ... and how you can too! / Sigrid de Castella

2nd ed.

Weight loss
Digestion
Nutrition
Obesity

613.712

Published by Andec Pty Ltd
PO Box 565 East Melbourne, Victoria 8002 Australia
For further information about orders: Phone 1300 925 215 or email: info@andec.biz

Cover Make-Up:	Jasmine Harradine - jasmine.harradine@gmail.com
Cover Photography:	Jayne Moberley - moberley.jayne@gmail.com
Hair Stylist:	David Sibilla - (+613) 9499 6677

Note: The photographs in this book have not been retouched other than cropping, lightening shadows and
removing backgrounds.

To my grandmother,
Esther,
one of the most courageous women I've ever known

A Personal Message from Sigrid

Dear friend,

Whether you're in Australia, or somewhere overseas, you are very special to me. You have given me a chance to inspire you to change your life for the better. And through that process you're also helping me spread my message across the globe to help reverse the world's obesity epidemic.

So I hope my book provides you with all the answers you've been seeking, so you can to reclaim your life, and enjoy all the natural good health, freedom and happiness you deserve … and be an inspiration to others too!

But the success of your weight loss journey depends on your participation. With the rise of social media apps, like Facebook and Instagram, the world has become a much smaller place. So I really hope you get involved with my *Half The Woman I Was* on-line community. You'll find all the links on the next page.

I look forward to meeting you soon, and to reading about your fantastic results!

Much love,

Sigrid

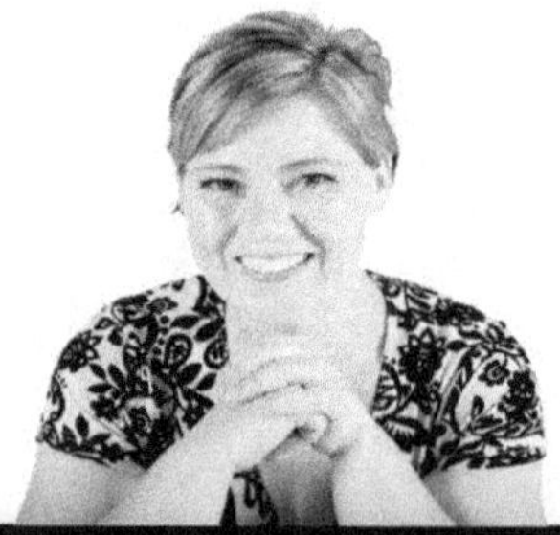

P.S. Don't forget to claim your $3,019 worth of VIP gifts that come with this book. Simply check the back of this book to get your password and login to the Members area of my website. I'll see you there.

halfthewomaniwas.com

instagram.com/halfthewomaniwasoz

facebook.com/HalfTheWomanIWas

twitter.com/HTWIW

pinterest.com.au/decastella

plus.google.com/u/4/+SigriddeCastella

youtube.com/user/HalfTheWomanIWas

Acknowledgements

There are so many people that deserve a thank you here - so many to whom I am so very grateful they could not possibly all fit here. To every person I have met, known or worked with in my life, I want you to know there is something undeniably inspirational about you - whether you know it or not. To be surrounded by your inspiration is a blessing for me, and for that I will be eternally grateful. Please accept my heartfelt thanks.

There are a few people close to me whom I would like to give extra special thanks – without them this book would not have been possible.

To my publishers - for believing in my vision and encouraging me on this journey. To my wonderful and supportive mother, Ros, for proof reading under impossible deadlines and coming through with the goods.

To Jayne Moberley for her amazing photographic skills, much love. And great thanks to Jasmine, Liz and David for working their styling 'magic'. To Marg de Castella, Hayley Barker, Tony Nolan and Geli Hangartner for their friendship, support and volunteering to handle my book launch.

To my nieces, Natasha and Rachel, for being there to look after our home and our fur babies when we travel, and for keeping me updated with stories and photos so I can relax, knowing they're in safe hands.

To "Aunty" Grace Chee for your friendship, support, nurturing and being there as back up fur baby sitter. I couldn't ask for anyone to love our 'kids' any more than you do. And I'm looking forward to more 'girl' time together.

To Ruth Watson, Frank Febo and Michael Kaltenbaugh for your unwavering friendship and support over the years, and for our many journeys together. True friendship is a gift – you are so special to me and I treasure our friendships so very much.

To my "brains trust" and dear BFFs Mikaela Smith-Chandler, Michelle Chant, Aubrey Perry, Nicola Barnard Gormley, Belinda Matchett, Catherine Grauf and Mel Campbell - thank you for your steadfast support and being there whenever I need you. Your friendships are irreplaceable, and mean more to me than I can possibly say.

To Dr Tracy Kopp, Daniel Seaton, Emily Hanscamp, Dr Georgina Whiting and Cindy Marr for keeping my body-mind connection strong, handling my physical ailments, and guiding me with your gentle and supportive care with humour and compassion.

To my parents Ros and Paul for raising me, guiding me, loving me unconditionally and allowing me to become all that I can be – you've done an exceptional job. I couldn't have asked for better parents.

Lastly, to my darling husband, Antony Anderson, my Neil Armstrong, Tony Robbins and Richard Branson all in one, who has taken me to places I never would have dreamed and whose continued love and support makes me want to be a better person each and every day. I love you.

And to you, dear reader, for anonymously inspiring me to write this book in the hope it eventually reaches you.

Now it has.

For additional tools and resources
to help you reach your goals faster
head to the official website.

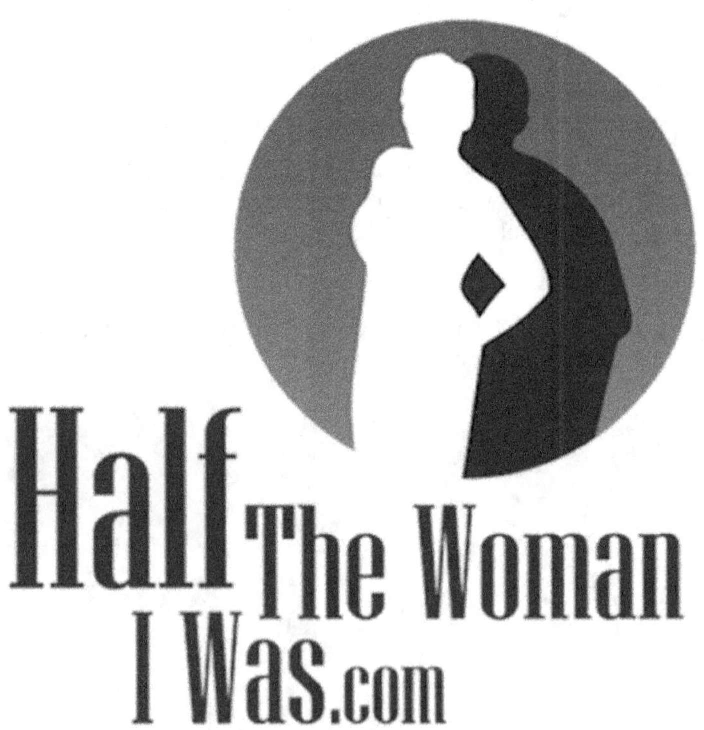

Table of Contents

Introduction

I grew up an obese child in a family of athletes. Running marathons was something that most of my family did regularly - or had done. Health and fitness was something that was valued incredibly highly, particularly as my uncle was an advocate of Nathan Pritikin. It was common to see him eat mung beans and sprouts when the rest us were eating more conventional but still very healthy food. As a result I always felt out of place in my family and, as I grew older and my weight increased, I felt more alienated, like I had been dropped into someone else's family of fitness freaks. In those days there were two things I knew for sure - there was no way I would ever run a marathon, and no way I would ever be thin. I was destined for a life of obesity with no way out.

As if being a fat child wasn't painful enough with all the teasing and name calling from the other kids, being a fatter adult was even worse. Having a famous surname synonymous with health and fitness, I was shamed almost every day as people who were introduced to me or saw the name on my credit card asked me if I was related to the Commonwealth Games Gold medallist. After replying in the affirmative I often felt their eyes gaze me up and down and silently ask the painful question "so why are you so fat?"

I truly didn't understand the reason, I just thought I was different. I believed I was born having inherited the world's worst metabolism. When I was very young my overweight mother had told me that, when she was pregnant, an endocrinologist who had tested her metabolism had remarked, "Well, there's good news and bad news. The good news is there is nothing wrong with you, but the bad news is you'd be the last person to die in a concentration camp and your children will grow into overweight people too". It was this story that underpinned my belief that no matter how hard I tried I was unable to lose weight. And I had lots of proof to support this belief. I had tried many times before to lose weight, but any temporary success of a few kilos would soon be reversed and I would weigh even more than before I'd started.

I desperately wanted to lose weight. When I daydreamed it was always as a thin person doing all the things I couldn't do. Nothing I tried had ever worked. Over the years I'd tried most diets - Weight Watchers, Herbal Life, Ayurvedic Body Type diet, Fit For Life, Eating Alive, Sandra Cabot's Body Type diet, the Blood Type diet, pills, and juices, Syndrome X diet, Detox, Atkins, Low GI, The Soup Diet, protein shakes, and the list goes on. Apart from not working for more than a couple of weeks (if at all) the only other thing that most of these diets had in common was they were just too difficult to manage, or I was hungry and un-satiated. The preparation time and restrictive nature was either too challenging to follow, or too difficult for my busy lifestyle. I kept searching for the answer, but my self-talk had convinced me there was none.

It was not until I was 34 years old and weighing in at more than 143kg (315 lbs) that I hit the wall and the answer to my lifelong problem revealed itself. It was only when I was ready, and willing to see, that the fog lifted and the 'Secret' was exposed. The solution was so fundamentally logical and technically brilliant that I couldn't believe no one had told me about it before. Actually I was really angry no one had. The honest truth is that this answer is in front of every person - if you are willing to see. Success and vitality is truly in everyone's reach - if you really want it. However the answer will remain hidden until you are truly ready, until you are willing to peel back the layers of your self-imposed cocoon of justification and remove your rose coloured glasses.

First and foremost what I had to understand was that no one could help me until I was ready to help myself. No matter how many people I asked for help, nothing was going to change until I was ready for the journey that would take me from obesity to health and vitality. That journey of 20 months in which I shed more than half of my body weight was done safely, naturally and without surgery. By gaining health and vitality I slashed years off my body age and added many more years to my life expectancy. I went from a size 30 to a size 10 and my feet shrank three full shoe sizes.

I was asked to write this book after many people who saw my transformation asked me what the 'Secret' was. My quick response to that question was "diet and exercise" but they will only get you half way there, if at all. The 'Secret' cannot be summed up in one or two sentences. I've tried many times, but it's just not possible. The 'Secret' is a holistic experience, so to sum it up in a few words neither does it justice nor explains the concept. To attempt to do so would misrepresent it and would prevent you from obtaining the results you've spent years yearning and searching for. The 'Secret' is a journey that each of us must take through self-education to knowledge and finally wisdom. This book is the ultimate distillation of all I learned in my journey from morbid obesity to health and vitality. If you devour each page as you would devour your favourite food then you'll learn the 'Secret' too and be able to put it into practice to achieve the result you've only ever dreamed of.

This book is not written for the skinny people out there that think they're fat when they're really not. You know the ones. This book is written specifically for the long term overweight and obese who are tired of being name called, ridiculed, discounted and rejected by a society that judges initially and largely on looks alone. This book is for those of you who now want to take control and change your life. I wrote this book to inspire you to achieve your health and vitality goals, no matter how many times you've tried (and perhaps failed) in the past. I know exactly how you feel – I was there. I can guarantee your life will be much more fun on this side of the fence and I'd love for you to join me.

There's a bumper sticker that says "I may be fat but you're ugly. I can lose weight". Remember all those people who caused you pain and use it for your motivation: success is the best revenge. Think about how jealous they'll be when you're at your goal weight looking absolutely fabulous. I can assure you they will be jealous, and you'll be the talk of the town (I was not only voted "most unrecognisable" at my 20 year high school reunion, but people were incredibly nice to me -even those that hadn't been nice or had ignored me at high school).

If there's one thing I have realised about the overweight and obese it's that they are generally incredibly capable and sensitive people, beautiful spirits. This is because they can't rely on their looks to be successful. Overweight people have to be far more competent, capable and connected than those who reply on their outer beauty. Whilst for those with a weight issue there may be little or no superficiality, there is usually a big brick wall that's hiding (and protecting) the light of their true spirit. I know there's a beautiful spirit inside of you - isn't it time you let it shine?

So now the real question is ... are you ready to join me in this journey? Are you tired of that excess weight you've been hauling around all these years? Are you ready to change your life and have everything you ever dreamed of? If the answer is "No", then thanks for reading so far and I wish you the best in life. If the answer is "Yes", even if you're completely petrified that it may all happen for you, or worse that it won't, then please read on. I'll be here to help you through, so hold on to your 'love handles' and be prepared for a journey that will challenge and rock your whole world.

Congratulations! In reading on you've already displayed some courage and commitment - you're awesome! Now a couple of things to mention before we start.

First, I have included literally thousands, of dollars of free bonuses in this book specifically to help you get real results. But I've deliberately scattered them throughout this book because most people only read the first couple of chapters and then give up. Or they read the summary at the end of each chapter and they miss the depth of meaning and full understanding, which means they then don't get the results they hoped they would. This is not that sort of book.

This book is a journey – it was my journey and now it's your journey. You'll get the most out of this book if you read it from beginning to end and do the exercises along the way. (And for those who really can't wait, the free bonuses are also listed on the back page of this book – check pages 270-1 for access details.)

The second thing is that truly nothing comes effortlessly, and it's exactly the same with this journey. I guarantee the road ahead won't always be easy. I guarantee at times the challenges ahead may even be quite painful. I guarantee along the way you will have doubts and you even may want to give up. But please don't - because I also guarantee that if you read this book cover to cover, do the exercises and incorporate the benefits of the free bonuses into your life then you will achieve everything you have dreamed of … and perhaps even more.

Now ... let's get going!

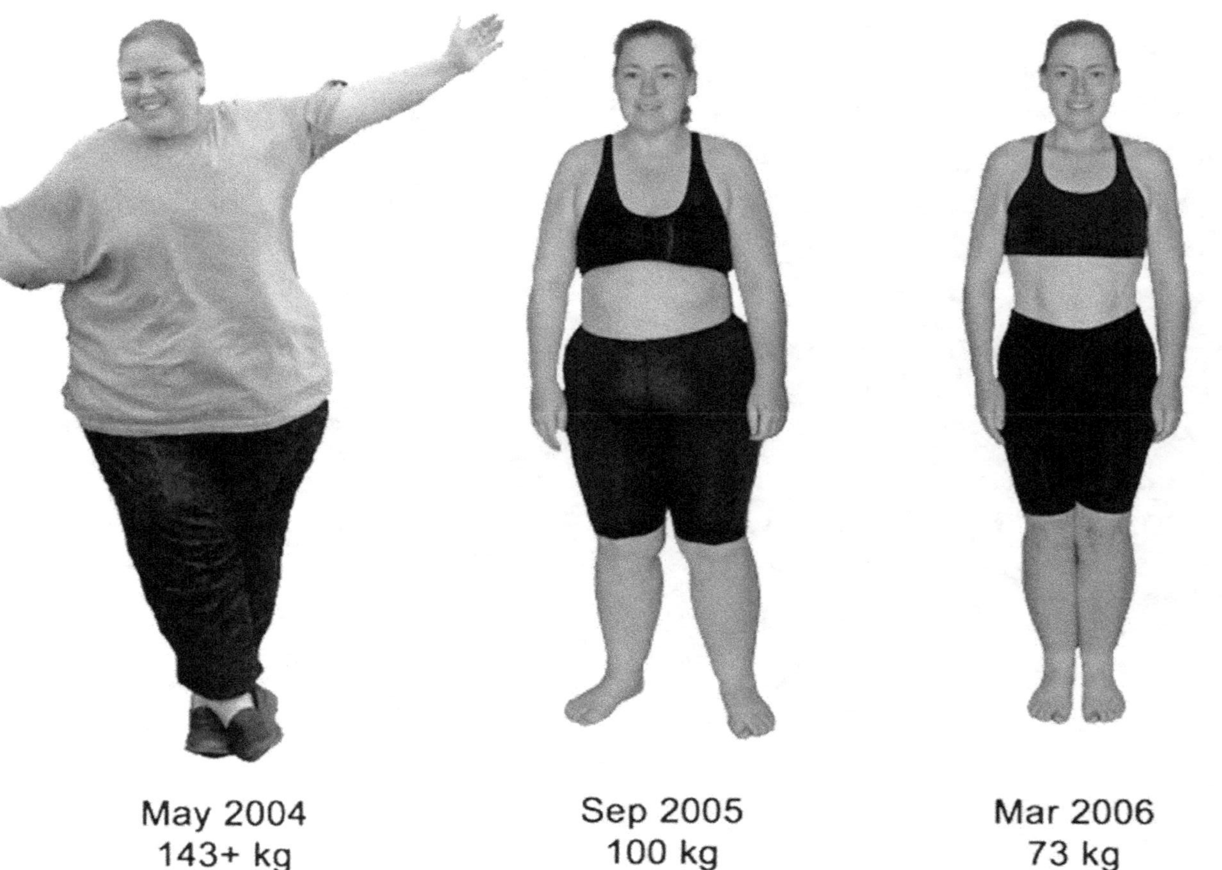
May 2004
143+ kg
Sep 2005
100 kg
Mar 2006
73 kg

Part 1:
Plan Your Trip

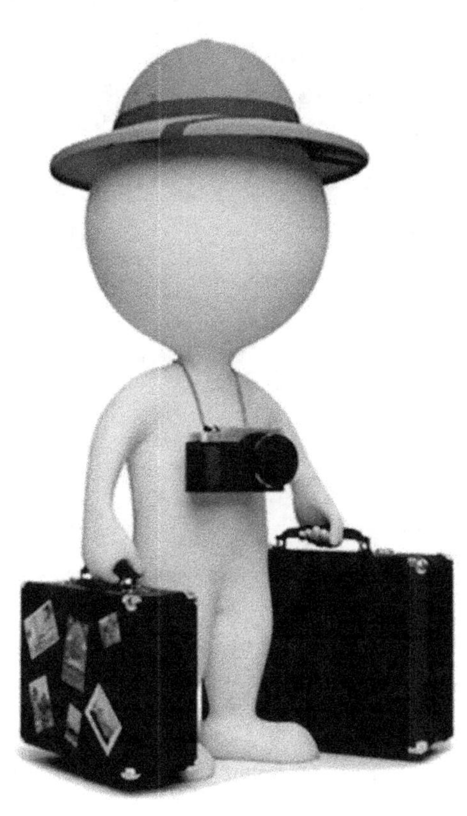

1. Overview

Welcome to the start of your journey and your new life. This book is divided into three parts: *Plan Your Trip, Your Itinerary and Reaching Your Destination.*

In this journey you're about to undertake I'll be your personal travel consultant who will help you plan for your trip, work out the right itinerary and give you the local knowledge relevant to each stop-over through to your final destination. More importantly I'll give you the tools and skills along the way, as well as a few handy travel gadgets, to make the journey easier, so you can become your own travel consultant for future journeys if you choose to take them.

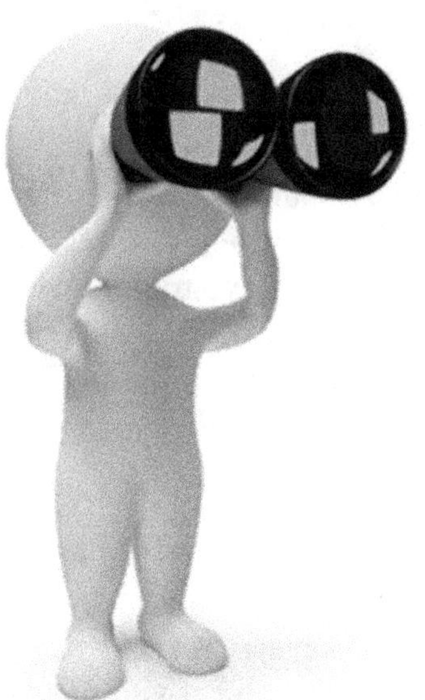

In Plan Your Trip together we'll be preparing the pre-travel plan for your journey - working out where you are right now and where your much desired destination is.

Your Itinerary will be divided into three sections: *Get Your Mind Right, Get Your Body Right* and *Get Your Spirit Right.* These sections are all about addressing each area of your being - Mind, Body and Spirit. Together we navigate the distant corners of your mind, body and spirit and bring them together to work as a single Itinerary to automatically support you in obtaining the results you desire.

In Reaching Your Destination together we'll explore your destination so you get the most out of being there, and we'll work out whether you're happy to holiday here for a while or where you want to go to next!

Most importantly, on this journey you'll be my **VIP**: Very Important Passenger, with exclusive and unrestricted access to all that I can share with you through this book and my **www.HalfTheWomanIWas.com** website. I've set a very special area aside for you on my website for all the extra stuff I couldn't cram into this book (check the last pages of this book for details).

Now, if you want to get the most out of this journey and get really great results then you need to do just two things.

The first is have fun. Okay, easier said than done, particularly when it's such a difficult, frustrating and sometimes painful subject matter like losing weight. Research indicates that you learn best and retain more information if you have fun at the same time. I have tried to write this book in a fun and informative style and I've enlisted the help of some little characters to give you a smile along the way. All I ask is that you try your hardest to try to have fun along the way. Give it a go. What do you have to lose?

The second is to participate fully. Your attitude determines your altitude. If you read this book with a "we'll see" or sarcastic "yeah, sure!" attitude, then you'll get little or average results. But if you're prepared to play 100%, full tilt, until you can't give any more, then your results will be incredible. If deep down inside yourself you don't really want your dreams, you don't truly believe in them, or they're not actually your goals to begin with, then you simply won't achieve them. Change your attitude and you'll change your results. Start right now to be fully engaged, participate 100% and take personal responsibility for your results. You'll be amazed how your life changes.

"If deep down inside yourself you don't really want your dreams, you don't truly believe in them, or they're not actually your goals to begin with, then you simply won't achieve them."

OK, so let's get planning. If you're ready and willing to have fun and participate fully then let's start by identifying where you're at now. Once we've done this then we can work out where you want to journey to.

2. Determine Your Point of Origin

First we need to work out where you're at now, your starting point, your origin. Without a starting point no course to your destination can be charted. For example, if you wanted to go and see the Eiffel Tower in Paris the exact path to get there is unknown unless you know where you're starting from. It's a relatively short journey if you're starting from Paris and a vastly different journey if you're starting out from Grand Central Station in New York City. Knowing your starting point will give you a clear understanding of the route you need to take.

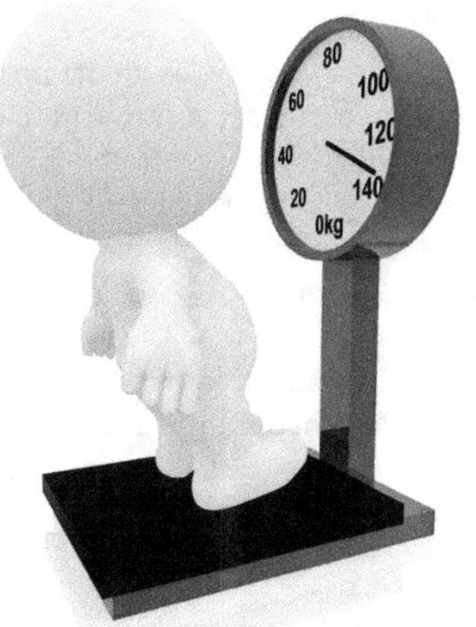

Starting out from Grand Central Station in New York City you would also realise the best way to get to Paris is by catching an aeroplane. So now you know it's going to be about a 12 hour journey and that you're going to need some resources along the way: your passport, some luggage, a guide book with a map of Paris and, to start off, some transport to JFK airport.

Understanding your starting point (origin), where you want to get to (destination) and knowing what things you'll need along the way (resources) is absolutely fundamental to preparing the plan for any journey (itinerary) and weight loss is no different.

What's important as you start this journey to better heath is understanding where you're at now, and how you got there in the first place. Often one of the most painful parts of any journey is facing the facts of where you are now – and usually this is because you're not where you really want to be.

> *"What's important as you start this journey to better heath is understanding where you're at now, and how you got there in the first place."*

My journey started with the horribly painful realisation that I could no longer measure how much I weighed because I overloaded the scales that were rated for 136kg (300 lbs) and measured up to 143kg (315lbs) before flashing with the big "OL" overloaded message. The fact is that I could have weighed much more than that (and probably did). But seeing that "OL" on the scales was a wake up call that I was on the fast track to disease and an early death. Facing this reality front on was embarrassing and painful because I had allowed myself to get to this position. I had no one else to blame. But I also knew that that my life was about to change and that from this point things would only get better.

Now it's time to record your current statistics and determine your origin.

In measuring your **weight** you need to a good set of reliable scales. At high weights the scales can become less accurate, so ensure the set you use are rated beyond your current weight and are a good set. Go to **www.HalfTheWomanIWas.com** and click on the **VIP** tab for my review of Body Fat Scales and recommendations.

It's best to weigh yourself ideally in the morning at your base weight (after you've fasted overnight), after you've been to the toilet and before you eat breakfast, or drink any fluids. It's important that you use the same scales each time you weigh yourself and that you always wear the same clothes, or none at all. Make sure your scales are used on a solid, firm, flat surface and never on an uneven or soft surface such as textured tiles or carpet. Record your results.

Measuring your own **height** can be a difficult task to accomplish, particularly by yourself. Not only is it hard to see what you are doing, you can easily measure it inaccurately. It's best to measure your height later in the day or after a full day of normal activities as the collapsible nature of the spine during overnight rest can make you up to a couple of centimetres shorter.

In measuring your height you need to take off shoes and any head gear (if you're prone to wearing hats). Grab a pencil and a small empty box at least five centimetres (2 inches) high. Stand on a hard surface (not carpet) as straight and as close to a wall corner or door jamb as possible. Stand with your back against the wall, feet together and with the back of your feet, bottom, shoulders, and the back of the head all touching the wall.

Look straight ahead, chin slightly tucked in, and raise the box above your head. Push the box against the wall so it's flat against the wall. Carefully slide the box down the wall until it gently rests on the top of your head. Holding the box firmly against the wall, carefully slide out from underneath the box, being sure not to move the box and use the pencil to mark the wall at the base of the box.

Use a measuring tape (preferably a metal builders tape) to measure from the floor to the pencil mark, ensuring your tape is as straight as possible by aligning it with the wall corner or door jamb. Record your results.

Measuring your **body fat** percentage at home is not possible without a good set of body fat scales. But if you have had your body fat professionally measured either at a gym or your doctor via scales or a set of fat callipers then record your result. If you can't access a regular measure of your percentage body fat then you can calculate your Body Mass Index (BMI) which will give you a rough idea of the range and category you're likely to be in. We'll discuss BMI's in the *Your Destination* section soon.

Measuring your own **blood pressure** is not really possible without a blood pressure machine. If you don't have one but you know your blood pressure or your doctor has recently measured it then record it.

It's important you get accurate body measurements by using a tape measure and keeping it taut to prevent sagging but not stretched (refer to the position diagram). Try to measure yourself in front of a full-length mirror so that you can see if the tape is positioned correctly. Keep your muscles relaxed while measuring and take all measurements from the same side of the body to ensure consistency. Stand up straight without shoes and with your feet 15 or 20cm (6 to 8 inches) apart unless otherwise stated, and record your results.

I prefer to measure unclothed, but you can also measure over properly-fitting undergarments or the thinnest clothes possible if this makes you more comfortable. Just ensure that anything you wear doesn't add to the measurements you take.

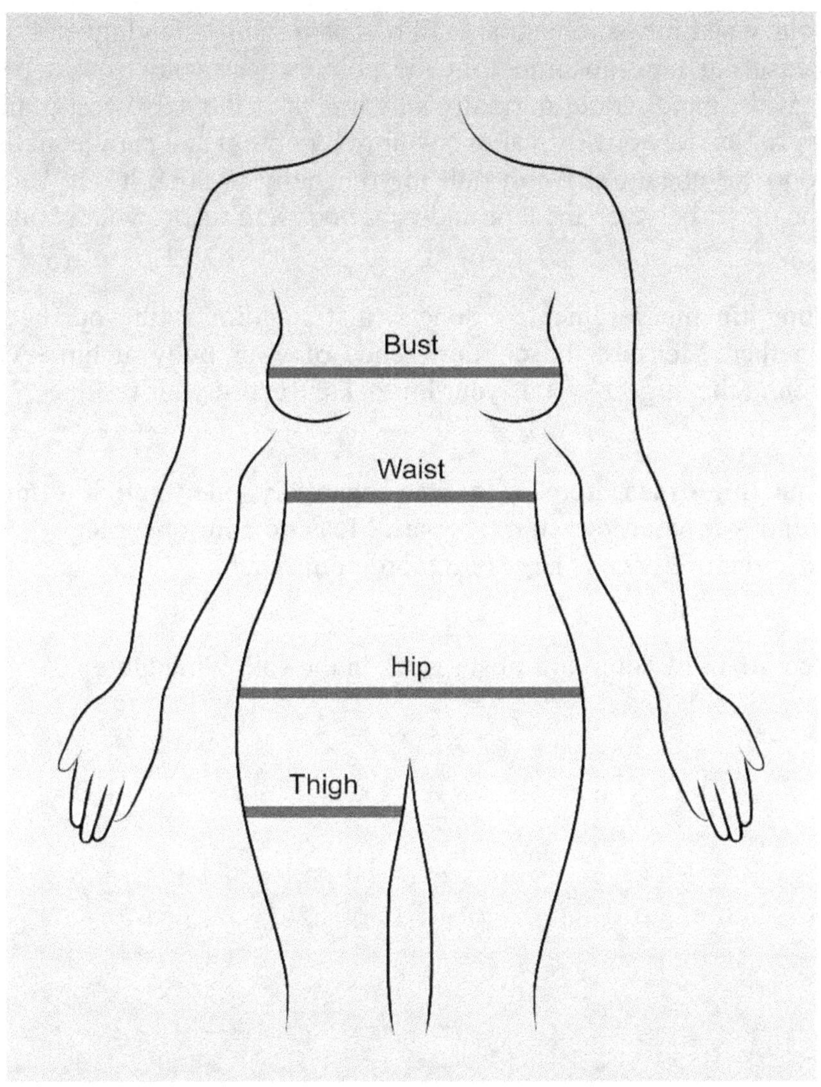

Your **chest** or **bust** measurement should be done while standing. Measure the fullest part of your chest, keeping the tape parallel to the floor and preferably with your arms relaxed at your sides (for this you can get a friend to help). Record your results.

Your **waist** measurement should be taken whilst standing and the measuring tape positioned at the point where your trouser belt or waist band would normally sit - this is at the narrowest point, approximately one inch above your belly button and parallel to the floor. No cheating! Don't pull in your belly or stick it out. Keep one finger between the tape and your body and record your results.

Your **hip** measurement is done whilst standing with your heels together. Measure the circumference of your body at hip level around the largest part of your buttocks. Record your results.

Your **thigh** measurement is done separately, one thigh at a time. Stand with your legs slightly apart. Measure your upper leg where the circumference is largest. Record your results.

Record all of your current statistics in the following table:

My Origin			
Weight (kg)		Chest (cm)	
Height (cm)		Waist (cm)	
Body Fat (%)		Hip (cm)	
Blood Pressure		Thighs (cm)	

What's Keeping You Here?

Okay let's face it. None of us want to weigh or measure everything we're eating, painstakingly write it into a diary and look every item up and painfully calculate our daily calories. It's boring and time consuming. I know because I did it for the first year of my weight loss transformation.

Computerised food diaries are much easier to manage, and, depending on what you eat, they can be relatively quick to use. Keeping a food diary quickly became my lifejacket for the first year, particularly because I discovered I was an over-eater. And keeping this diary provided me with a massively valuable education in nutritional values - I learned a lot along the way. Once I was able to re-educate myself and self-manage my food intake I was able to discard my lifejacket.

If you think you may need a lifejacket and use a food diary then go to **www.HalfTheWomanIWas.**com and click on the **VIP** tab for my review of Diet Diaries and my recommendations.

Food diary or not, working out how many calories you're consuming to keep at your current weight will give you a better idea of your potential to lose weight, which can be very encouraging information.

> *"Working out how many calories you're consuming to keep at your current weight will give you a better idea of your potential to lose weight."*

To find your maintenance level and the number of calories in foods, follow the steps below:

- Convert your current weight from kilograms to pounds by multiplying it by 2.21. e.g. 100 kilograms x 2.21 = 221.0

- Multiply your current weight in pounds by 15. This gives you your current maintenance level. e.g. 221 x 15 = 3315

So if you weigh 100 kilograms (221 pounds), then you're probably consuming around 3315 calories to keep you at that weight. And if you're exerting yourself physically and doing a lot of exercise then you're actually consuming far more.

So at over 143kg (316 pounds) I was actually consuming around 4700 calories (and I did compare this by measuring my intake via my food diary on a typical day and it was so accurate it was a little scary).

Obviously the first step is to reduce your calorie intake – this is a no-brainer, right? Duh! But most people go about this in the completely wrong manner and they stop losing weight after a week or so. Later on we'll discuss the right way to reduce your calories so your weight doesn't plateau even if you do no additional exercise. And the kicker is if you also increase your level of physical activity, even slightly, you'll lose even more. We'll continue exploring these themes in Chapter 3: *Decide On Your Destination*.

In determining your point of origin you also need to understand if there are any particular factors that led you to reach this place. Think about the choices you have made in your life, both good and not so good, that have led you here. Some of those choices have supported your goals, but some have not. For the most part you will instinctively know which ones were not the best decisions for you.

If you're wanting to explore more about how your choices and decisions effect your current situation then head to **www. HalfTheWomanIWas.com** and click on the **VIP** tab and take the *Lifestyle Profile Quiz*. You may find it quite revealing!

Key Learnings

What are the top three things you have learned about yourself in this chapter?

1. ____

____

2. ____

____

3. ____

____

Describe how you are feeling about your current situation?

____

____

____

____

Are you ready and willing to change? Why?

____

____

____

____

What are the top three changes you think you can make that will help you get to your destination?

1. ____

____

2. ____

____

3. ____

____

3. Decide On Your Destination

Now that you know your starting point and how you got here (your origin), you can decide on your goal (your destination) and why you want to get there.

Destination Weight

What's your ideal weight?

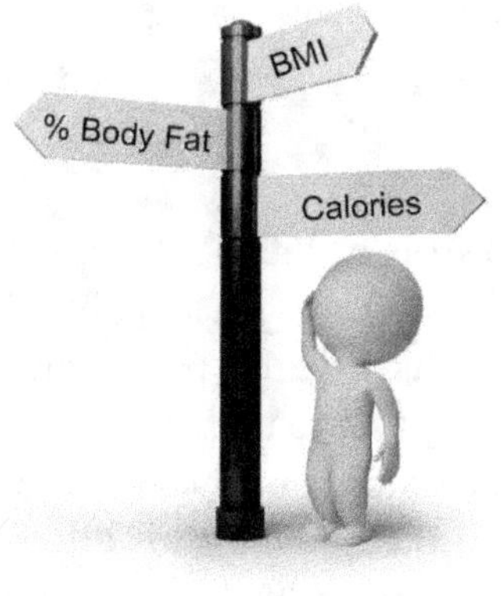

Those who grew up with a fairly normal body size will have an idea of what weight they were previously happy at, or what weight they would like to be. But if, like me, you've never been a healthy weight then working out your target weight can be very confusing. There are so many recommendations, opinions and calculators out there and most will give you vastly different results, with several weight recommendations seemingly bordering on the pursuit of anorexia.

And into the mix we can also throw another measurement – Body Mass Index (or BMI). BMI is a tool that's used a lot in the weight loss industry. Its calculation is derived from the individual's body weight divided by the square of his or her height. Most of us know that body weight is made up of lean muscle mass, organs, bones, fat, tissue and around 70% water. But it's important to understand that muscle weighs more than fat, so if you have a higher proportion of muscle in your body than the average person, your target weight for your height will be slightly higher than for someone with a lower proportion of muscle. This doesn't mean you are overweight for your height. This is one of the reasons that men, for their height, will generally weigh more than women - they develop muscle more easily due to the higher presence of the male hormone, testosterone.

> *"Muscle weighs more than fat!*
> *Muscly people tend to weigh more but this doesn't*
> *mean they're overweight for their height."*

BMI is a statistical measurement based on averages and it does tend to skew what is reasonably achievable at both ends of the height scale. This results in taller people having a BMI that is uncharacteristically high compared to their actual body fat levels. It also does not take into account the amount of muscle mass in a body, which weighs more than fat. So the BMI index tends to overestimate the amount of body fat for people who are naturally more muscular, body builders, high performance athletes and pregnant women. Equally the index tends to underestimate the amount of body fat for the elderly and people who have a disability or wasting disease. And it doesn't provide an accurate measurement for people with eating disorders like anorexia nervosa or those with extreme obesity.

Simplistically BMI is not a very accurate measurement for people outside the 'normal' range. Having said all that, it is a good guide in conjunction with other measurements to understand your current situation. Most countries have a similar BMI's ranges to Australia's which is as follows:

BMI Range	Category
< 20	Underweight
20-25	Healthy Range
25-30	Over Weight
30-35	Grossly Over Weight
> 35	Obese

If you're not sure what a healthy weight is for your height then go to **www.HalfTheWomanIWas.com** and click on the **VIP** tab for my *Complete Body Calculator* for assessing BMI and your ideal weight.

Decide now what weight you would ideally like to be. And don't forget, you can always revise your weight as you get closer to your goal if need be. For me my first goal was 100kg (220lbs). Once I'd reached it I then felt comfortable and confident enough to reset my goal to 72kg (158lbs). Write your target weight down now as closely as you feel comfortable to your ultimate goal.

My Destination Weight (kg) is:

Destination Calorie Intake

Now we need to determine your target calorie intake so we can compare it with your current calorie intake. Using the same formula in Chapter 2, calculate your target calorie intake:

- If you're starting in kilograms then convert your target weight from kilograms to pounds by multiplying it by 2.21. e.g. 70 kilograms x 2.21 = 154.7

- If you're starting in stones and pounds, then convert this to total pounds. e.g. 11 stone 1 pound is 11 stone x 14 pounds, plus 1 pound = 155

- Multiply your target weight in pounds by 15. This gives you your future maintenance level. e.g. 154.7 x 15 = 2320

So for me it looked like this:

Current Daily Calorie Intake:	4700
Destination Daily Calorie Intake:	2320
Target Daily Reduction:	2380

When you see this completed for your own scenario be warned you may get a shock. I didn't realise I was actually consuming more than twice the amount of calories I needed for my goal weight (which made sense as I was twice the size!) Even if your Target Daily Reduction value is not twice, it may be large enough to freak you out: "Oh my goodness I'm eating how many calories?", or "Gosh, how on earth can I survive on half the amount of food?"

Don't freak out. The good news is you won't have to.

First, we start the transition slowly by reducing your calorie intake by a meagre 200 calories per day. This is a small change you won't really notice. It's a large enough change to make a difference, but small enough to fool your body that nothing has changed. Next, you stay at that slightly lowered calorie limit for a minimum of two weeks, preferably a month or until you feel ready to move to the next lower level. You are in control of this change, you are the pilot flying your own plane to your own exotic destination.

You should plan to lose not more than one kilogram (2.2 pounds) a week. More than that means you are shocking your body and throwing it into starvation mode, which will slow your metabolism and that's when things go wrong. Taking small steps and progressing slowly means the weight will come off, and it'll stay off. The reality is it probably took you years to get to the weight you are (it took me over 30 years!) and so you can't realistically expect for things to change overnight – it will take time.

> *"It probably took you years to get to the weight you are*
> *... you can't expect things to change overnight."*

And there are plenty of other changes to be made that will support this small reduction in having a huge effect on your progress. We'll discuss this in Chapter 6: *Get Your Mind Right.*

Record your results below.

My Current Daily Calorie Intake is:

My Destination Daily Calorie Intake is:

My Daily Target Calorie Reduction is:

Destination Body Fat

Weight measurements in conjunction with body fat percentage are the most accurate measures of your progress so it's helpful if you can incorporate body fat measurements into your plan.

Fat deposits itself on the body in different areas depending on a range of factors including gender, genetics and age. The percentage of essential body fat, the level below which physical and physiological health would be negatively affected, is 2% to 5% in men and 10% to 13% in women.

The most reliable measurement for body fat is via hydrostatic or underwater weighing, however this is not very convenient and is not a readily available process. Fortunately now you can easily determine your percentage body fat with the use of a good brand of body fat scales.

Body fat scales use a technique called Bioelectrical Impedance Analysis (BIA) to measure bone density, by passing a small and completely harmless electrical current through your body. The scales then use a formula to calculate body fat based on body density. However there is no one formula fits all and differences in age, gender, ethnicity, body size, and fitness level all have a significant effect on the results, as does your body position, the amount of water in your body, your food intake, skin temperature and recent physical activity.

So make sure you find the right set of scales that can be calibrated as closely as possible to your situation. Scales that allow individual setting for adults/children, men/women and height can help to more accurately predict results. And don't skimp – accuracy will almost certainly increase with price. As previously mentioned there are some great body fat scales around that are not too expensive. Head to **www.HalfTheWomanIWas.com** and click on the **VIP** tab for my *Review of Body Fat Scales* and my recommendations.

However accurate or inaccurate the result, what is important in this journey is that you use the same set of scales to monitor your progress over time. Don't compare it too closely with tables or the results of family or friends. What's important in using a set of body fat scales is that you standardise each measurement.

You can do this by:

- Measuring yourself at the same time of day for each test

- Making sure your water / fluid consumption (or lack thereof) is the same before each test, or alternatively drinking the same amount one hour before each test

- Not measuring yourself after exercising as this affects hydration levels

- Trying to ensure the room temperature is the same each time to reduce the effect of skin temperature on the electrical current used by the scales

- Cleaning the foot plates with an alcohol swab and drying them off before each test

"Use the same set of scales to monitor your progress and standardise your measurements."

If you do not have access to a set of reliable body fat scales then you can use a body fat calculator to approximate the percentage fat in your body. Visit **www.HalfTheWomanIWas.com** and click on the **VIP** tab to access my *Complete Body Calculator*.

Determine what your body fat percentage is now, and where you'd ideally like it to be according to the following table:

Type	Women	Men
Essential Fat	10–13%	2–5%
Athletes	14–20%	6–13%
Fitness	21–24%	14–18%
Average	25–31%	18–24%
Obese	32%+	25%+

From the table above decide on the type of body you'd like to achieve and determine the right destination percentage body fat that's right for you.

My Destination % Body Fat is:

Destination Blood Pressure

Blood pressure is the pressure circulating blood exerts on the blood vessel walls. Blood pressure varies and comprises of two measurements:

the diastolic (minimum) and the systolic (maximum) pressure.

Blood pressure results are influenced by heart rate, blood volume, viscosity of the blood and resistance caused by the diameter of the blood vessels. The average blood pressure in (mmHg) for the following age groups is:

1 Year	6–9 Years	Adults
95 / 65	100 / 65	110 / 65 – 140 / 90

Blood pressure is also influenced by physiological factors including stress, alcohol, drugs, diet, exercise, obesity and disease. As these conditions improve or reduce many people find elevated blood pressures begin to return to the normal range.

Blood pressure monitors are relatively inexpensive and it can be good to monitor your blood pressure particularly if, as I do, you suffer from 'white coat hypertension', so called because some patients exhibit elevated blood pressure in a clinical setting, but not in other non-clinical settings such as when they self-administer the test at home.

My Destination Blood Pressure is: /

Destination Measurements

You may have a dream of being a gorgeous Marilyn Monroe-esque 36 – 23 – 37 inches but at only 1.66 metres (5ft 5in) tall metres her weight varied between an anorexic 53kg (116 lbs) to a healthier 63kg (138 lbs). The reality is that if you're anything other than an hourglass shape this is probably not going to be achievable, no matter how hard you try.

So in considering your target weight you should not only consider your height, BMI and body fat percentage, you should also consider your body shape and consider destination measurements that are in alignment with your natural body shape.

"Your target body measurements need to be in alignment with your natural body shape."

Women are broadly categorised into four main geometric body shapes, although there are very wide ranges of actual sizes within each shape. The shapes are banana, apple, pear and hourglass.

The most common shape for women is **"banana"** – 46% of women are more straight or rectangular in body shape. Waist measurements are usually between 0 cm to 22 cm (0 to 8.6 inches) less than the hip or bust measurement. For "banana" women fat tends to accumulate in the abdomen, buttocks, chest, and face.

Just under 14% of women are **"apple"** shaped and tend to resemble an upside-down triangle with broader shoulders and bust, and narrower hips. "Apple" women have a tendency for slim legs and thighs and an out of proportion abdomen and chest compared to the rest of the body. For "apple" women fat is distributed predominately in the abdomen, chest, and face.

Around 20% of women are **"pear"** shaped, more closely resembling a regular upward triangle, traditional pear shape, spoon or bell. "Pear" women have a hip measurement that is greater than their bust measurements. For 'pear' women fat tends to be distributed around the waist and upper abdomen, with a tendency for a generous rear, full thighs, and a smaller bust.

Less than 8% of women closely resemble the **"hourglass"** shape – the traditional image of female beauty and desirability. Hip and bust measurement are often almost equal with a smaller narrower waist. For "hourglass" women fat tends to accumulate around both the upper body and lower body, enlarging the arms, chest, hips, and rear before other parts, like the waist and upper abdomen.

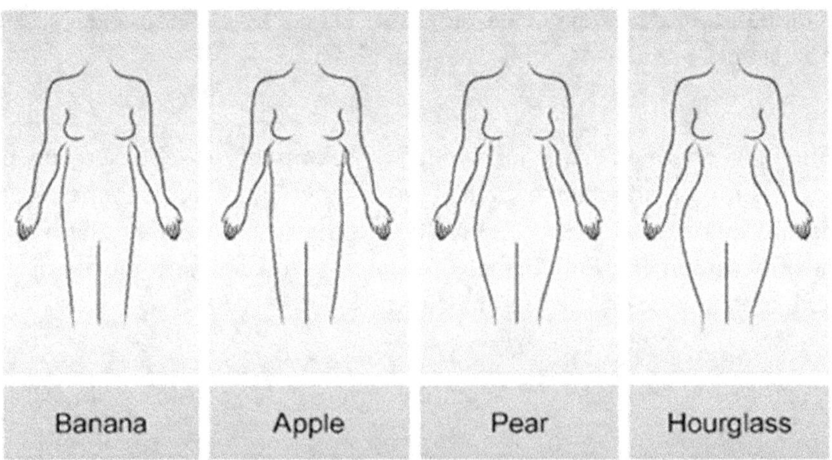

I am decidedly a pear with my hips being much wider than my relatively tiny waist.

Keeping your body shape in mind, if you've never been a small size before, you may like to refer to the following Australian Women's Size chart for a guide to what your measurements could be.

Australian Standard Size Chart - Women				
Size	Bust (in cm)	Waist (in cm)	Hips (in cm)	Pant Length (in cm)
6	81	58	87	104
8	86	63	92	104
10	91	68	97	105
12	96	73	102	105
14	101	78	107	106
16	106	83	112	106
18	111	88	117	107
20	116	93	122	107
22	121	98	127	108
24	126	103	132	108
26	131	108	137	110

This chart is in centimetres. So to convert the measurements to inches divide each number by 2.54.

After all this, if you're not sure what body shape type you have, or what your measurements could be then simply head to **www. HalfTheWomanIWas.com** and click on the **VIP** tab to access my *Complete Body Calculator*.

Otherwise write down your goals now:

My body shape is:	Apple	Banana	Pear	Hourglass
My Destination Chest Measurement is:				
My Destination Waist Measurement is:				
My Destination Hip Measurement is:				
My Destination Thigh Measurement is:				

Additional Indicators

There are a number of other health indicators that might be helpful in your journey - there are literally hundreds of pathology tests available. Depending on your current circumstances, risk profile and aims it may be worth measuring your starting position for a range of testable health factors.

Some of the more common tests are listed below for consideration.

FBE / FBC / Full Blood Picture: This is one of the most commonly ordered tests and provides valuable information about the kinds and numbers of cells in the blood: red blood cells, white blood cells and platelets. Abnormalities in any of these types of cells can indicate the presence of a medical disorder including anaemia or viral infections like glandular fever.

U and E's / Urea and Electrolytes: This test is used to determine kidney function and whether there is a problem with the body's electrolyte balance, which is the various salts in the bloodstream including sodium, potassium, chloride and bicarbonate.

LFT / Liver Function Tests: There are 7 different tests that may be used to detect liver damage: ALT, ALP, AST, total bilirubin, albumin, GGT and total protein, but they all basically reveal if any liver enzyme levels have risen. Up to five of the tests are measured at the same time on one blood sample.

TG /TRIG / Triglyceride; Blood / Total Cholesterol; and other blood lipid levels: Tests used to determine the risk of heart disease by finding out the levels of both HDL-cholesterol, LDL-cholesterol, total cholesterol and triglyceride levels.

Glucose / Blood Sugar / Blood Glucose / BSL, OGTT, GTT: This test checks whether your blood glucose levels are within a normal range, or whether they are elevated indicating diabetes, or lowered indicating hypoglycaemia.

To get an indication of the tests you should consider go to **www. HalfTheWomanIWas.com** and click on the **VIP** tab to complete your *Medical Risk Profile* and then refer to your doctor who will work out with you which tests are right for your personal circumstances.

A quick word on disease and medical conditions: Many of you may have present a disease or debilitating condition you have had to learn to live with. These conditions can get you down. But it is possible to reverse many of these conditions and reduce or eliminate the symptoms. I have hereditary lymphedema – a condition (in my case genetic) that causes localised fluid retention and tissue swelling. This is thought to occur due to poorly developed or missing lymph nodes in the body and it can be quite debilitating and painful. Whilst my condition, thankfully, is only grade 1 and mild, as a child this condition added to my bulk and made it difficult to exercise, thereby adding to my weight problems.

During my journey I found that if I walked regularly, ate right, drank lots of water and slept with my legs slightly elevated I could reduce my swelling immensely and cease any need for diuretics or other medication. Losing the weight and changing my diet has further reduced the severity of my condition. Even so, I still have to be careful how long I sit without walking around as it only takes an hour or two before my legs start to swell and can become painful.

If you have a condition that is restricting you from achieving your goals please know that the changes you will make on this journey may well bring you more relief than you could have imagined. If I'd said I wasn't going to walk because it was too painful then I may never have discovered that walking brings me immense relief.

Whatever the changes you choose to make, if you have a medical condition please use your common sense and consider whether you should discuss these changes with your doctor prior to making them.

> *"Remember to discuss any proposed changes with your doctor prior to implementing them."*

If you think that there are additional indicators for testing that may be of particular use for you then please write them down now.

My Additional Destination Indicators are:

Travel Duration

How long it takes to reach your destination depends on your point of origin and your individual goals. Whatever your goals don't expect to lose weight too rapidly. Weight loss is sustainable and permanent only when it's lost slowly at a recommended average of no more than 1kg (2.2 lbs) per week.

Be aware that any radical change in diet or exercise will yield a huge weight loss in the first week, and a reduced but still relatively large weight loss in the second week. However over time your weight loss rate per week will reduce and flatten out to an average amount – some weeks you will lose nothing at all. This can sometimes lead to feelings of failure or that the new regime is not working. This is not necessarily the case and it's important that you stay true to your regime and follow the plan. The weight will continue to come of gradually, and stay off.

Allow a week for every 0.8 of a kilogram (1.7 pounds) you want to lose – if you lose it faster then that's okay, just don't push your body too fast as it will rebel! Calculate your travel duration by dividing the kilograms you want to lose by 0.8, or total pounds by 1.7. For example if you want to lose 20kg (44 lbs) safely and permanently it will take at least 25 weeks (half a year!)

> *"Permanent weight loss is about losing weight slowly, so allow at least one week for every 0.8kg (1.7 lbs) you want to lose."*

Visit **www.HalfTheWomanIWas.com** and click on the **VIP** tab to access my *Complete Body Calculator* to understand how long it will take to get to your ideal weight.

Record your results below.

My Travel Duration is: weeks

Key Learnings:

Now put all the information from Chapters 2 and 3 together and complete the following table:

Summary			
My Origin		**My Destination**	
Height (cm)		Height (cm)	
Weight (kg)		Weight (kg)	
Body Fat %		Body Fat %	
BMI		BMI	
Blood Pressure	/	Blood Pressure	/
Daily Calorie Intake		Daily Calorie Intake	
Additional Indicators to consider:			
My minimum Travel Duration is:			Weeks

What are the top three things you have learned about yourself in this chapter?

1. ____

____

2. ____

____

3. ____

____

Describe how you are feeling about your goals and destination?

____

____

____

____

Describe how you are feeling about taking this impending journey?

____

____

____

____

What are the top three changes you think you can make that will help you get to your destination?

1. ___________________________________

____

2. ___________________________________

____

3. ___________________________________

____

4. Pre-Travel Preparation

Before you begin your journey there are some things you need to prepare. Having a 'clean sweep' of your environment will help support you to stay on your new path to success.

Exercise 1: Remove Temptation

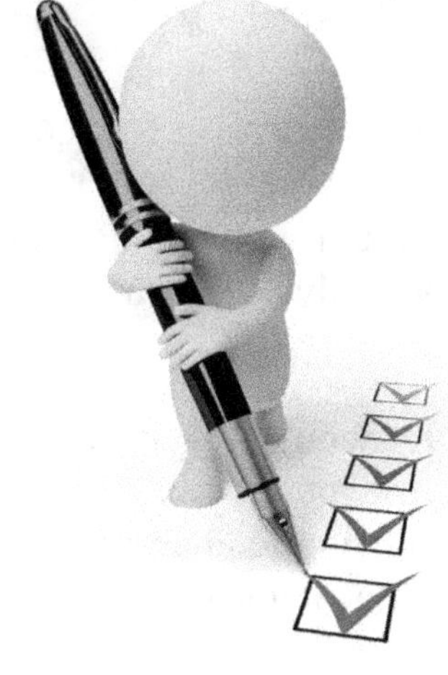

In preparing for this journey it's critical that you remove all unnecessary temptation from your environment. This will ensure you don't slip back into old the old eating habits that got you into your current state. You'll need at least an hour to perform this exercise.

Start by cleaning out your pantry and fridge of all high sugar and refined foods. Check the ingredients on your packed, canned and frozen goods carefully. If you see the ingredient sugar, high fructose corn syrup, or any word ending in 'ose' (e.g. maltose, dextrose, fructose, etc.) then ditch it. Check the *Understanding Nutrition* section for more names for unhealthy sugars in *Get Your Mind Right*.

You should also remove the following foods: potatoes and potato-based products, white rice, wheat, white bread and foods containing baker's flour (this will likely also include wholemeal bread). Also review all your processed and packaged foods – foods lose their nutritional value during processing so most processed foods have little or no nutritional value. Check the ingredients on each pack and if there's more than a couple, or they sound 'chemical', or you can't pronounce it, chances are it's not going to provide any real nutritional benefit and isn't good for you.

> *"Get rid of all processed and low nutrition foods and those high in sugar and fat so they won't tempt you."*

If you're not 100% sure whether you should ditch it or keep it, keep it until you've read the *Get Your Mind Right* section after which you'll have a clearer understanding of whether it's good for you or not (and you'll probably end up ditching it!)

Don't fret about throwing all this food out – it's got no good nutritional value for anyone and shouldn't be consumed. But if you have a real issue about throwing food away then donate or gift your unopened goods to someone you know will use them.

Exercise 2: Pack Your Bags

Now it's time to consider the rest of your environment and how it can support you better. Your environment is really a true reflection of yourself, so if your life isn't going quite the way you want it to, starting with a spring clean of your environment can help turn things around.

Your Wardrobe:

Let's move to the bedroom ... open your closet and look in your chest of drawers. How many clothing items are in there that you no longer fit into? Usually it's a lot! Don't worry, we're not going to throw anything out yet.

You'll need to set aside a couple of hours for this task and you may need a friend to help you, particularly if you're a bit of a hoarder and have trouble throwing things out (and don't worry, we'll be working on that issue in a later section).

Go through your closet and chest of drawers and remove every item that either doesn't fit you, or that you never want to wear again and place it on your bed into three piles:

1) the things you really want to fit back in to;

2) the things you really want to fit back into but know that you really never will, and;

3) the things that should have been thrown out years ago because you'll never wear them again (you know ... that tie died t-shirt you bought in Bali, those 70's flared corduroy trousers and that glo-mesh top). Don't forget to go through your shoes too.

Get some large garbage bags (or vacuum storage bags). Piles 1 and 2 are to "keep" but the items will be kept in storage until you are in a position to wear them. Pile 3 is the "ditch it" pile that can either be donated to charity or thrown away.

Put the "keep" items in a storage cupboard (not your closet) or preferably in the garage. What should be left are only the clothes you can wear at the moment. Whilst this is a difficult task to complete (admitting you no longer fit into some of your favourite clothes) it will be liberating once done.

For years every time you opened your closet to decide what to wear you were confronted with the shame and the guilt of all those clothes you can no longer fit into. And it also made choosing something to wear a time consuming event. Now, when you open your closet you will only be able to select clothes that you fit into. No shame, no guilt and quicker decision making.

As these clothes get looser, you can bring out the bags in storage and add some of them to your closet, provided you fit into them and still want to wear them. Chances are you'll want a new look as you become thinner and may not want them after all.

> *"Your environment is a true reflection of yourself - just like a mirror."*

Spring Clean Your Environment:

Getting your house in order is just as important as getting your body, mind and spirit in order.

In the bedroom start by reviewing your bed linen – are your sheets threadbare and old? If so throw them out and get yourself a nice new set of sheets, preferably made of cotton or natural fibres so they can breathe. There is nothing as sublime as sleeping on high thread count quality linen – I used to be happy with 'Red Circle Boutique" sheets but now I'm a fully converted 1000 count girl!

Make sure your bed pillows are in good condition and are the kind to provide the correct support to your head and neck. What about your mattress or futon? To get the most out of your sleep periods select a mattress or futon made from organic cotton, wool, or latex, and ensure it has the right support for your body type. Your mattress and pillows should be replaced every five years to ensure adequate support and hygiene. When was yours last replaced?

Now about that clutter – nick-nacks everywhere, clothes not put away? Everything in the bedroom should have its place. If it doesn't and you can't find a valid reason for it being there then get rid of it or put it back where it should be. Oh and one last thing, no eating in the bedroom – ever!

You actually spend quite a bit of time in the bathroom (and the toilet). How's the hygiene level? Does it need a spring clean? Any ugly black mould anywhere? Is your bathroom littered with all sorts of half used make up, expired medicines and dozens of little bottles of hotel shampoo, conditioner and bath gels? What about all those hair clips, scrunchies, hair gels and sprays? Time for a clean out and rationalisation – and perhaps a new shower curtain.

If your towels are old and tatty then it's time for a new set – get a full set of bath sheets or luxurious large towels, hand towel, bath mat and face washer. And while you're at it get a new toothbrush if you haven't replaced yours in the last three months.

Is your laundry piling up, ironing not done? If your clothes aren't wash and wear (which is all I try to buy these days) then outsource your ironing. Ironing ladies aren't expensive and you'll feel great that all your clothes are ready to wear at a moment's notice.

Do you have dozens of appliances in the kitchen, none of which you use because you hate cooking? Most of us have appliances that are not supportive of our dietary habits – so give away or sell that waffle maker and deep fryer. Hang onto the grills and steamers. And if you really want to do yourself a favour get rid of all your appliances and invest in a Thermomix – the health benefits and ease of cooking is really worth the investment. And what about your crockery, glasses and cutlery? Are they chipped, broken or bent? If so replace them.

There's a few things we need to attend to in the lounge room. First things first, put away all those DVDs and hide the TV guide. Watching TV is going to keep you sedentary and is not going to help you burn that fat. Having said that it can be a good distraction from exercise. So if you a have an exercise bike, treadmill, orbital trainer or something similar then you can put that into the lounge room and watch your favourite shows while you work out. If you don't have a piece of exercise equipment then you can hire one!

To get the most out of your eating plan it's important to eat each meal at the dining table (not in front of the TV) - eating is about ritual. During your journey you'll need to re-educate your body and establish a new ritual – that eating should be done slowly and enjoyably. For your dining table buy a special place mat, napkin, and a special place setting for one – one plate, one bowl, once glass, one set of cutlery. It doesn't have to be expensive, just something you like. Sitting down to a fresh meal with your new setting, turning some spa-style music on and eating slowly, putting your knife and fork down between mouthfuls and chewing each mouthful at least 10 times before swallowing will give you a whole new outlook, and will also give your body enough time to register it's eaten so you eat less.

> *"Create an eating ritual ~ eat slowly and enjoyably
> at the table and not in front of the TV."*

Do you have a study or spare room? Is it a well organised space or is it a dumping ground for things you don't know what to do with but don't want to get rid of? If you can't face cleaning this room out (and would rather shut the door) then at least stack everything up neatly so you can enter the room. As you gain strength and confidence this is one room that you just may be up for tackling. Consider converting your unwanted items into extra cash by selling them.

And don't forget to change your light bulbs. Fluorescent lights and energy saving globes gradually dim over time and the globe you once thought was bright may now be leaving you in the dark. Low light levels and a lack of sunshine can lead to Seasonal Affective Disorder (SAD) or winter depression, making you tired, over eat, crave carbohydrates and have a tendency to withdraw from the world and hibernate (which just makes things worse). By changing your globes to daylight rated LEDs (check the maximum allowed on your light fittings and lamps) you'll not only see more, but your mood will also rise. In one of my companies I replaced the four year old fluorescent office and factory lighting with high intensity day-light fluorescents. Not only was it so bright it felt like working in the Bahamas, the mood of every staff member lifted dramatically, absenteeism went down and productivity and profit both rose.

Spring cleaning shouldn't be restricted to the inside of your home. Around the house get rid of unwanted rubbish or broken items, ensure the lawn is regularly mown and the garden beds weeded. Planting a few colourful annuals near the front door in water reservoir pots can also brighten your home and make you feel much better without requiring a lot of attention. Gardening is good exercise but if you are time poor then hire someone else to do it for you.

You may sometimes feel you live in your car, and as it gets you from A to B when you need it to, doesn't it also deserve a clean? Get rid of all the rubbish, the empty food wrappers and drink bottles, discarded clothing, extra pair of shoes, newspapers and magazines. Getting your car washed and waxed outside and cleaned inside doesn't take a lot of your energy or time, or cost a lot of money. And while you're at it, is your car overdue for a service?

As you may be starting to realise there are many facets to the very necessary task of getting your house in order so that not only your mind, but also your environment supports you in your goal of weight loss.

Are you up to date with your tax returns? Do you have a financial plan? Have you written a will? Do you have adequate house insurance, health insurance, life insurance, trauma and income protection?

If not then go see your accountant, financial planner, lawyer or insurance broker. And if you have overdue debts or credit cards contact your financial institutions and make payment arrangements – you'll be amazed at how flexible they will be if you proactively make new arrangements and stick to them. The bottom line is that addressing these matters is important to clearing the noise from your life so you can concentrate on the journey you're about to take.

> *"Spring clean all facets of your life ~*
> *clear the noise from your life so you can*
> *concentrate on the journey you're about to take."*

At work, rather than getting bogged down by the day to day activity and tasks that are seemingly urgent and important (but really aren't), take a few hours out to clear your desk of the clutter and reorganise your files. And set aside time at the end of each day to plan and prioritise the next day's activities rather than just lurching from crisis to crisis. You'll be so much more productive and will reclaim valuable hours.

I understand that the sheer thought of all there is to do here may be completely overwhelming and enough to make you go and reach for the Tim Tams®! For complete and permanent results you have to make a total commitment to your goal, not just tinker around the edges. Remember you can always throw some money at the problem and outsource! For additional help to tackle these items visit **www.HalfTheWomanIWas. com** and click on the **VIP** tab to access the *Resources Directory* for contacts and special offers.

Exercise 3: Analyse Your Time

The final exercise before you head off on your journey is to determine your daily schedule. The biggest excuse for people not exercising or eating correctly is they don't have time. So we're going to focus on removing unnecessary activities and streamlining your day, so you can fit more of the 'right' stuff in.

First, write down what you typically do each hour on a weekday and for each day of the weekend.

It may go something like this:

	Time	Weekday Activity	Saturday Activity	Sunday Activity
AM	1:00	Sleep	Sleep	Sleep
	2:00			
	3:00			
	4:00			
	5:00			
	6:00			
	7:00	Wake up, shower, dress, breakfast		
	8:00	Travel to work		
	9:00	Work	Wake up, Shower, dress, breakfast	
	10:00			
	11:00		Housework	Wake up, Shower, dress, breakfast
PM	12:00	Lunch Out		R&R time
	1:00	Work	Shopping	Snack
	2:00		Shopping / take away lunch	R&R time
	3:00		Work	
	4:00		Shopping	
	5:00			Snack
	6:00	Drinks after work	Unpack shopping	R&R time
	7:00	Travel home		
	8:00	Dinner in front of TV	Dinner out with friends	Dinner in front of TV
	9:00	R&R time		R&R time
	10:00		Bar with friend	
	11:00	Sleep		Sleep
AM	12:00		Travel home, Tv, sleep	

You can see in the above example schedule that this person spends a lot of time socialising, eating out and lots of usually unproductive R&R time (which they may spend watching TV, reading, playing on the Internet or generally mooching around, particularly on Sundays after a long sleep in). You may also notice that there seems to be no regular physical activity.

In reviewing your current schedule, you need to determine if your activities are going to be supportive of achieving your goals. Ask yourself whether the activities are:

1) core to your life, that is, your own self-maintenance (e.g. sleep, work, eating, etc.) or if they are

2) leisure or pleasure activities that are optional and able to be moved, compressed or reworked (e.g. watching TV, socialising, etc.).

Now rework your table but add whether the activities are Core or Optional (Opt).

	Time	Weekday Activity	Core	Saturday Activity	Core	Sunday Activity	Core
AM	1:00						
	2:00						
	3:00	Sleep	Yes				
	4:00						Yes
	5:00			Sleep	Yes		
	6:00					Sleep	
	7:00	Wake up, shower, dress, breakfast	Yes				
	8:00	Travel to work	Yes		Opt		
	9:00			Wake up, shower, dress, breakfast	Yes		Opt
	10:00	Work	Yes		Yes		
	11:00			Housework		Wake up, shower, dress, breakfast	Yes
PM	12:00	Lunch Out	Yes		Opt	R&R time	Opt
	1:00			Shopping	Opt	Lunch or Snack	Yes
	2:00	Work	Yes	Shopping / take away lunch	Opt		
	3:00				Yes	R&R time	Opt
	4:00			Shopping			
	5:00				Opt	Snack	Opt
	6:00	Drinks after work	Opt	Unpack shopping	Yes		
	7:00	Travel home	Yes			R&R time	Opt
	8:00	Dinner in front of TV	Yes	Dinner out with friends	Opt	Dinner in front of TV	Yes
	9:00	R&R time	Opt			R&R time	Opt
	10:00			Bar with friend	Opt		
	11:00						
AM	12:00	Sleep	Yes	Travel home, TV, sleep	Opt	Sleep	Yes

Now that you've completed the table and tagged all items Core or Opt, we need to focus on the Core activities. Add up all the hours in a week for the items you've tagged Core.

Deduct this number from 168 and this will give you the maximum number of hours possible to put towards goal achievement, if you so choose.

For example:

Weekday Activity	Core	Hours	Saturday Activity	Core	Hours	Sunday Activity	Core	Hours
Sleep	Yes	8	Sleep	Yes	8	Sleep	Yes	10
Wake Up, shower, dress, breakfast	Yes	1	Wake Up, shower, dress, breakfast	Yes	1	Wake Up, shower, dress, breakfast	Yes	1
Travel	Yes	2	Housework	Yes	2	Meals	Yes	2
Meals	Yes	2	Shopping / Unpack	Yes	3			
			Meals	Yes	2			
Sub-Total Core Hours		13	Sub-Total Core Hours		16	Sub-Total Core Hours		13

Weekdays (5 x 13)	65
Saturday	16
Sunday	13
Total Core Hours PW	94
Hours in a Week	168
Maximum Hours Available	74

In the above schedule there are a maximum of 74 hours available to put towards goal-related activities. This is over 10 hours per day on average. Think of what you could do with all this time. And even if we deduct the standard 40-hour work week, it still leaves 34 hours at least!

Now the reality is that you may be a busier person than this example. You may have kids or elderly parents to look after, you may do some volunteer work or you may work more than 40 hours per week. And you're still going to want to go out with your friends, you're still going to want to watch some TV or read or mooch around the house. But this example, although it may be extreme, shows that for most people, finding a couple of hours a day is more than possible. And this is without maximising your core activities, like taking your lunch to work for a 30 minute break rather than eating out and taking an hour.

There are lots of tricks you can do to maximise your core hours and fit in goal-related activities by multi-tasking. We'll explore more of those ideas soon. But for now what is important is you realise that many of the things you're doing now are just filling up your time, and they're not contributing to your goals.

> *"Many of the things you're doing now*
> *are just filling up your time ~*
> *they're not actually contributing to your goals."*

In fact, a lot of the activities you undertake are actually preventing you from achieving your goals. The question is, are you going to continue to let this happen?

If the answer to that question is "No" then start taking control of your life by finding at least two hours per day to commit to goal-related activities, that's a total of 14 hours per week. You may wish to do more on the weekend, that's your choice. But all I ask is you commit at least two hours per day (other than reading or performing the exercises in this book) to regaining your health and vitality.

If you want to do a more thorough analysis of your time then visit **www.HalfTheWomanIWas.com** and click on the **VIP** tab to access the *Personal Scheduler Tool.*

Exercise 4: Prepare Your Daily Schedule

Now that you've worked out the blocks of time in your day available for goal-related activities draw up a schedule, stick it to your fridge and follow it!

It may go something like this:

	Time	Weekday Activity	Saturday Activity	Sunday Activity
AM	1:00	Sleep	Sleep	Sleep
	2:00			
	3:00			
	4:00			
	5:00			
	6:00	Wake Up Goal Oriented Activity 1hr		
	7:00	Shower, dress, breakfast		
	8:00	Travel to work	Wake Up Goal Oriented Activity 1hr	Wake Up, shower, dress, breakfast
	9:00	Work	Goal Oriented Activity	R&R time
	10:00		Shower, dress, breakfast	
	11:00		Housework	
PM	12:00	Bring Lunch / 30 mins break		
	1:00	Work	Lunch - Home	Lunch - Home
	2:00		Shopping	Goal Oriented Activity
	3:00			
	4:00		Unpack Shopping	
	5:00		Shopping	
	6:00	Travel home	R&R time	R&R time
	7:00	Dinner - Home		
	8:00	Goal Oriented Activity	Dinner out with friends	Dinner - Home
	9:00	R&R time		R&R time
	10:00		Travel Home / Sleep	
	11:00	Sleep		Sleep
AM	12:00		Sleep	

This is an example of a more balanced week with time for socialising, R&R, plenty of sleep and 16 hours of goal-related activity each week.

Once you've worked out your rough plan on paper, go to **www. HalfTheWomanIWas.com** and click on the **VIP** tab to access the *Personal Scheduler Tool* to create your official weekly plan.

Key Learnings

What are the top three things you have learned about yourself in this chapter?

1. _______________________________________

____

2. _______________________________________

____

3. _______________________________________

____

Describe how you are feeling about removing temptation from your life and clearing out your environment?

____

____

____

____

What are the top three temptations you need to remove?

1. ______________________________

____

2. ______________________________

____

3. ______________________________

____

What are the top three areas you need to clean out in your environment?

1. _______________________________________

____

2. _______________________________________

____

3. _______________________________________

____

Describe how you are feeling about your time analysis?

____

____

____

____

What are the top three changes that you can make to your daily routine to increase your time?

1. ____

____

2. ____

____

3. ____

____

Part 2:
Your Itinerary

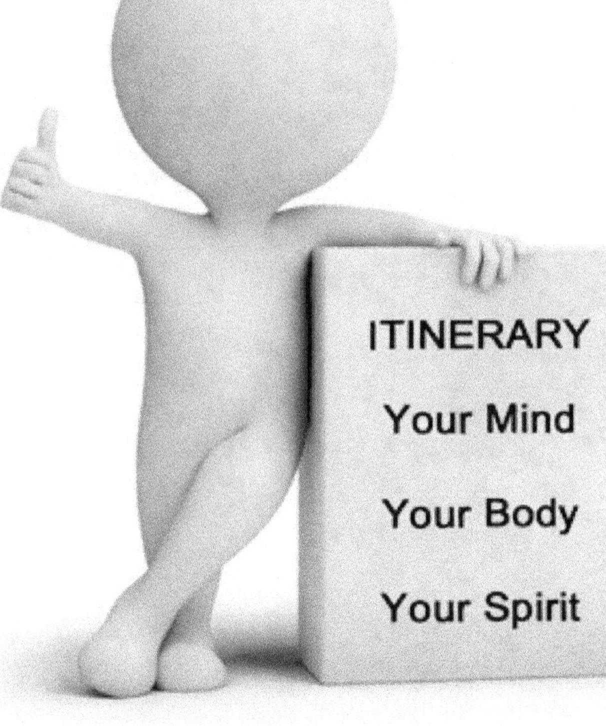

5. Create Your Itinerary

With your point of origin and your destination now identified, the next step is to create your personalised itinerary.

An itinerary can be defined as the proposed outline of a journey, a travel diary or guidebook. This section is just that – it's your travel bible that will provide all the help and support you need to get you from your point of origin to your destination.

For the purpose of this journey, your itinerary is divided into three sections: *Get Your Mind Right; Get Your Body Right*; and *Get Your Spirit Right*.

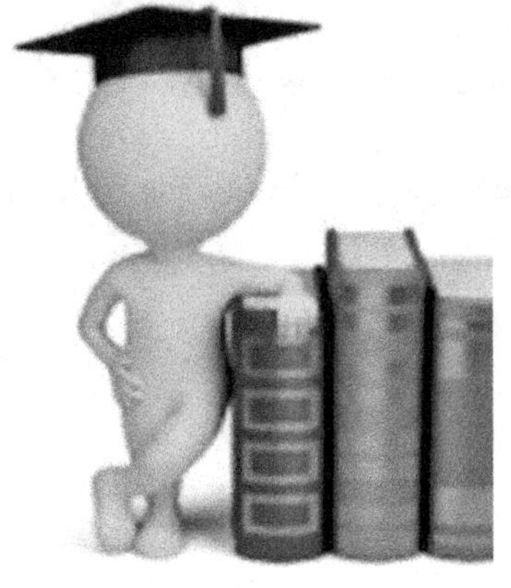

In *Get Your Mind Right* we'll be working on your knowledge base. You'll gain an understanding of why diets don't work and you'll learn all about nutrition – from amino acids to zinc and everything in between. You'll gain an understanding of why the body needs each and every one of these components as well as the recommended daily intakes and best natural sources. You'll find out whether supplements work, or whether they're just burning a hole in your wallet. We'll discuss hydration and what it really means. And you'll learn ways to control your portion sizes.

In *Get Your Body Right* we'll be working through the physical requirements of the body, and how to increase activity safely and sensibly. You'll learn the best forms of exercise to burn up your fat stores. You'll also gain an understanding of your metabolism and the 16 techniques you can use to speed it up. We'll discuss how stress is linked to weight gain, and you'll learn how to nurture and love your body so it supports you in getting to your destination.

Lastly, in *Get Your Spirit Right* we'll discover the qualities and skills required of any Captain in chartering their own vessel. You'll discover what sort of Captain you are, and where you need to improve. Together we'll explore how aligned the parts of your mind are (or are not) and what you can do to bring everything you've learned together to make your journey easier than you could have possibly dreamed.

By following this three-step Itinerary you can virtually be assured of reaching your destination safely, on time and on budget. Before we get started you need to set your intention for this section. Please share your thoughts for the things you'd like to achieve from each of the next three areas by completing the following questions.

What are the top three things you hope to learn from *Get Your Mind Right?*

1. ____

   ____

2. ____

   ____

3. ____

   ____

What are the top three things you hope to learn from *Get Your Body Right?*

1. _______________________________

____

2. _______________________________

____

3. _______________________________

____

What are the top three things you hope to learn from *Get Your Spirit Right?*

1. _______________________________________

____

2. _______________________________________

____

3. _______________________________________

____

Thanks for sharing. Now let's get going!

6. Get Your Mind Right

Why Diets Don't Work

What do you think of when you hear the word diet? Calorie restriction, mood swings, starvation, hunger, rabbit food? Over time the understanding of the word diet has been skewed to negatively mean to restrict oneself to small amounts or special kinds of food in order to lose weight.

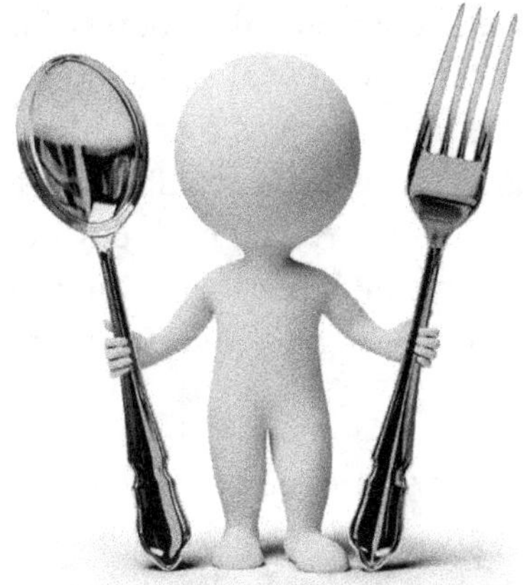

However the word diet is actually a noun meaning the type of food that a person, animal, or community regularly eats – something we all do whether the food is good for us or not. The word diet should not have a negative connotation, or a positive one for that matter. It just is what we do every day in the consumption of food to support life.

Unfortunately many people have decided to live to eat, rather than eat to live. For most of us the quantity of food we eat is greater than we require, and the quality of food readily available to us has decreased considerably.

But let's look at what happens when we go on a conventional "diet" or fad diet, where the intake of calories is restricted in order to lose weight.

Why do we lose so much weight in the first couple of weeks? What happens in our bodies and why do we stop losing weight after that?

In the first couple of weeks our body is operating according to the prior instructions we gave it where there was an overabundance of high calorie, high fat foods and no scarcity, no famine - eat anything you want at any time. So the body generally has a high metabolism and is burning a high rate of calories; in fact obese people generally have higher metabolisms than skinny people.

But after the first few days the reduced calorie intake slows the metabolism and the body swings into starvation mode. It actually adapts to the lower level of calories by lowering your basal metabolic rate so you don't burn as many calories as you were previously. To continue to lose weight you would need to continue to reduce calorie intake (and increase exercise) each day or two and eventually, taken to the extreme, you would be eating nothing each day, that's if your body didn't collapse and your organs shut down first!

When you place your body on a calorie restricted diet your body actually begins to eat itself and, as muscle is easier to convert to energy that fat, your body begins to waste away and your percentage of lean muscle mass (the bit that actually helps you lose weight) drops, leaving you still with the fat you were trying to get rid of in the first place.

On top of that, when people go on a restricted eating plan the shift in the type of foods they consume is usually quite radical. They swap highly processed and refined packaged food full of tasty salt, sugar and fat (not to mention artificial flavours and colours) for healthy options of fruit, vegetables and lean meats. The body has been used to all those additives and, like a junkie, the body continues to crave those additives for several weeks until they have been completely voided from the system.

> *"Fad diets don't work and continuous dieting is one of the worst things we can do to our body."*

Enter into this equation the mental aspect of "giving up" those foods packed with additives that we associate with enjoyment and all of a sudden your mood swings and depression hits. Couple this with the usual lethargy and tiredness one experiences and it's a recipe for disaster. And don't forget the self-inflicted isolation. Food is a huge part of our social interaction – meal times are often spent with family, friends or colleagues. Often when we go on a restricted eating plan we also hibernate and reduce the number of social outings that involve food in order to remove temptation. But this also isolates us and makes us feel worse.

So what's the end result? We end up breaking or cheating on our diet because it's not sustainable. Days, weeks or months later we try it again and the result is the yo-yo diet cycle of losing weight, gaining it back plus a little more, losing, and gaining again. Yo-yo diets not only place a huge amount of stress on the body and its systems, it's mentally very stressful and weakens your immune system making you more susceptible to sickness.

All these self-inflicted aspects of a reduced calorie intake lead us into creating and carrying with us negative feelings toward healthier "diet" foods. Plus they create such powerful negative thoughts around restricted eating plans that even if they did work, our subconscious would ensure we'd fail. We'll discuss more about this concept in Chapter 8: *Get Your Spirit Right*.

Now that I can reflect on my emotional state at my highest weight, I seemed happy but was actually quite depressed. Desperate to find a 'quick fix' to my problem I seriously considered that stomach stapling may be the cure. However after investigating it on the Internet and seeing the premiere of the US series The Biggest Loser I slowly became convinced that more natural methods were preferable and so commenced my self-education in nutrition. Before you make any radical changes to your lifestyle I'd like to share with you what I learned.

Understanding Nutrition

Processed foods lack nutrition and may fill you up temporarily, but they don't provide the vitamins and minerals your body needs to maintain optimal health. This eating plan is all about getting back to basics – mostly fresh fruit and vegetables and lean meats, but also some selected nuts and grains.

Whilst nothing eaten in small quantities is taboo, you should for the most part avoid all processed foods, white coloured carbohydrates (with the exception of small quantities of brown rice and whole rye bread), and avoid all sugars and the 'bad' and 'ugly' fats. Alcohol (which is a sugar) is also best minimised.

You may have heard of this approach before, but what makes this plan so special is the education around the physical (food and exercise) and the metaphysical (spiritual and subconscious) components. As you continue reading you will begin to understand how all of these components work together to produce a whole, which is the observable you. When they are aligned and in synergy you will get the results you desire. When they are not aligned your health is suffering.

Look in the mirror.

Are you where you want to be?

How is your lack of understanding or misunderstanding of nutrition affecting your body?

In the following sections we will be looking at all aspects of nutrition broken down into their component parts. For each part we'll consider its importance to the body, the Recommended Daily Intake (RDI) for adults, diseases and ailments arising from deficiency or too much (toxicity) and where you can find the best natural sources of each.

This next section is rather long (and possibly a bit bland or repetitive for some) but it's really important in gaining an understanding of what happens in your body. So please don't skip it, keep reading.

PROTEIN

Importance:	Macronutrient used for the building and repair of body tissues, producing enzymes, hormones, and other substances the body uses.
Deficiency Diseases:	Marasmus and Kwashiorkor
RDI Adult:	0.75 to 1 gram per kilogram of body weight**
Toxicity Risk:	Over consumption may be associated with weight gain, intestinal issues and kidney problems from the inability to process by products.
Best Natural Sources:	Meat, seafood, dairy and eggs. Vegetarians and Vegans should increase their consumption of nuts, quinoa, oats, chickpeas and tahini.

** The amount of protein required in a person's diet is determined in large part by overall energy intake, the body's need for nitrogen and essential amino acids, body weight and composition, rate of growth in the individual, physical activity level, individual's energy and carbohydrate intake, as well as the presence of illness or injury.

The Good, the Bad and the Ugly

What makes a protein good or not is its nutrient base, omega-3 fatty acid value, saturated fat value and how it was raised, grown, farmed, stored and treated before it's cooked. Biodynamic meats are very good, but they become ugly very quickly if you fry them in oil.

Soy-based products are packed with nutrients and can be a good substitute for vegans and vegetarians and those with lactose intolerance. However soya contains phytochemicals and phytoestrogen, which are great for women undergoing menopause, but not so great for the average person. So having too much soya can have hormone-altering side effects. I remember when I found out I was lactose intolerant I switched to soy everything (milk, cheese, ice cream), consumed too much and it wasn't long before my face broke out in really nasty boils – I couldn't leave the house for two days!

The Good:	Beans, legumes and lentils, lean low fat, low salt meats (grill or poach), egg whites and soy products in moderation.
The Bad and the Ugly:	Those that are high in saturated fat, contain virtually no nutrients and high levels of salt like full fat processed meats, bacon and over marbled steaks.
Healthy Tip:	Trim all meat and fish of fat and skin and only grill or poach where possible.

CARBOHYDRATES

Importance: Macronutrient used to provide energy to the body.

Deficiency Diseases: Excessive liver ketones, abnormal fat metabolism, breakdown of body protein, increased sodium excretion, loss of energy and fatigue.

RDI Adult: 45% to 65% of daily calorie intake

Toxicity Risk: Nil

Best Natural Sources: Raw, natural vegetables, fruits, grains and legumes.

The Good: Complex carbohydrates are molecules that the body must digest very slowly and so they have a low and gradual impact on blood sugar levels. There are three types: glycogen, starch and fibre (soluble and insoluble).

Glycogen is found in glucose, which is stored in the liver not in food. Starch is found in rice, grains and some vegetables (like potato). Fibre is found in fruits, vegetables, grains and legumes and may be soluble (absorbed by the body such as oats, fruit and vegetables) or insoluble (passes unabsorbed through the digestive tract such as nuts, seeds, and whole grains).

The Bad and the Ugly:

Simple carbohydrates are molecules that the body is able to digest and convert to sugar/energy very quickly - they have a rapid impact on blood sugar levels. There are two types: monosaccharides (glucose, fructose and galactose) and disaccharides (sucrose, lactose and maltose).

Healthy Tip:

Aim to consume carbohydrates in their raw or natural (low GI) form, and cook them as least as possible. The processing of carbohydrates increases their Glycaemic Index (the speed at which they convert to sugar in the body). So home-boiled brown rice is best as are raw rolled oats not porridge mixes.

I am a self-confessed carbohydrate addict. I love breads, the white fluffy ones that have no food value as well as artisan sourdoughs. But I have had to learn to avoid as many simple carbohydrates as possible and substitute flours for paleo ingredients and eat paleo 'breads' instead.

FAT

Importance:
Macronutrient used to provide energy, build healthy cells, make hormones, help with the uptake of vitamins A, D, E and K and provide healthier skin.

Deficiency Diseases:
Fatty acid deficiency, dermatitis, joint problems, menstruation problems, fatigue and poor brain function.

RDI Adult:
65g total fat (of which no more than 20g is saturated fatty acids) in a 2000 calorie diet.

Toxicity Risk:
Too much fat or the wrong kind can lead to "fat cell toxicity" where the fat cells produce toxic hormones (adipokines) that increase blood pressure, blood clotting, inflammation and insulin resistance leading to cardiac issues, diabetes and other problems.

Best Natural Sources:
Fish (particularly salmon), shellfish, flaxseed (linseed), hemp oil, chia seeds, pumpkin seeds, sunflower seeds, leafy vegetables, walnuts, avocado and olive oil.

The Good:
Triglycerides (fats and oils) as unsaturated fats (excluding trans fats) that consist of monounsaturated fats and polyunsaturated

fats and are usually a liquid at room temperature. Monounsaturated fats are found in olive oil, avocados, nuts and seeds. Polyunsaturated fats can be found in foods such as oily fish (sardines and tuna), soy beans and walnuts.

Another good fat is phospholipids, the double layer of fat that surrounds all cells in the body to keep them healthy. The richest source of phospholipids is lecithin which can be found in eggs, liver, peanuts, soy beans and wheat germ.

Sterols are important for producing many hormones, vitamin D and for making cholesterol. They are found in plant food as phytosterols and in animal food as cholesterol. Both these types of sterols generally have a healthy impact with the exclusion of LDL cholesterol (as found in fatty cuts of meat and animal brains), which should be avoided to ensure good cardiovascular health.

Essential fatty acids are fats that the body cannot make on its own (unlike cholesterol that it makes) but daily intake is required to produce prostaglandins that regulate many body functions. These fats are Omega 3 and Omega 6.

The Bad and the Ugly: Triglycerides (fats and oils) as saturated fats, and trans fats are both bad fats. Trans fats occur during the manufacturing of processed foods via the hydrogenation of vegetables (e.g. cakes, biscuits, etc.) and are also found naturally in smaller amounts in ruminant animal foods. All these fats negatively impact the body's health by increasing the risk of cardiovascular disease.

It's best to also avoid soy products like soy (or soybean) oil (which adversely affects hormone levels and possibly causes heart disease), as well as canola (rapeseed) oil which is predominately made from genetically modified plants and produced using chemical solvents.

Getting The Good Oil

Many oils change their chemical composition when heated, and an oil that was good for you at room temperature can quickly become bad for you. Due to its high caloric value, minimising the use of oil is important and buying good non-stick cookware will reduce your need to use it in the first place. There are some health concerns with Canola and Vegetable oil (which contains Canola), and palm and coconut oils are very high in saturated fats and should be avoided. So if you do need to use oil here's a guide to the better ones to use in moderation.

Almond Oil: high in monounsaturated fat low in saturated fat
Taste: nice nutty flavour
Best used: at room temperature - should not be heated

Avocado Oil:
High in monounsaturated fat, low in polyunsaturated fat and packed with vitamins A, D, E, and B-group
Taste: mild flavour, green in colour
Best used: at room temperature - should not be heated

Grapeseed Oil:
High in polyunsaturated fat, lowers bad LDL cholesterol and raises good HDL cholesterol and is a rich source of vitamin E
Taste: light, pleasant
Best used: at room temperature or for low to medium heat

Macadamia Oil:
High in monounsaturated fat and low in polyunsaturated fat
Taste: nutty with some aftertaste
Best used: at room temperature or for low heat cooking

Mustardseed Oil:
Good balance of omega-3 and omega-6 fatty acids and has a very low saturated fat content
Taste: Strong, can overpower foods
Best used: at room temperature or for low heat cooking

Olive Oil:

Monounsaturated fat

Taste: light and pleasant to strong and robust depending on grade and pressing

Best used: at room temperature or for low heat cooking

Peanut Oil:

Monounsaturated but higher in saturated fat. Those with nut allergies should avoid this oil.

Taste: distinctively nutty and can overpower non-Asian dishes

Best used: at room temperature and for low to very high heat cooking

Rice Bran Oil:

High in saturated fat but free of trans fats

Taste: virtually none

Best used: at room temperature and for all cooking including frying (not that you should be doing any) due to its incredibly high smoke point

Sunflower Oil:

Polyunsaturated monounsaturated, both help reduce cholesterol levels

Taste: light and works well with most foods

Best used: at room temperature for low to high heat cooking

FIBRE

Importance:	A complex carbohydrate with little food value, important for aiding digestion, reducing the risk of colon cancer, lowering cholesterol and assisting with diabetes.
Deficiency Diseases:	None, however low levels may result in constipation and increased risk of colon cancer.
RDI Adult:	30 – 45g
Toxicity Risk:	Nil
Best Natural Sources:	Raw fruits, vegetables, grains and cooked legumes.
The Good:	There are two types and five components of fibre (pectin, cellulose, hemicellulose, lignin and gums).
	Soluble fibre dissolves in water and is digestible. Rich sources are fruits (pectin) and legumes.
	Insoluble fibre does not dissolve in water and is not digestible but promotes regular bowel movements and prevents constipation. Rich sources are vegetables

(cellulose, hemicellulose and lignin) and grains.

The Bad and the Ugly:	Whilst there is no bad fibre, gums and thickeners are a type of fibre that is generally used as a food additive in processed foods, and as such this type of fibre is not recommended.

SALT (also see Sodium)

Importance: Required by all living things to regulate the body's fluid balance. Sodium also assists with electrical signalling of the nervous system.

Deficiency Diseases: Rare but low sodium levels can lead to muscle cramps, dizziness and electrolyte disturbance.

RDI Adult: 1150 to 5750 milligrams of salt which equates to 460 to 2300 milligrams of sodium.

Toxicity Risk: High consumption of salt can lead to high blood pressure, stroke, edema, stomach cancer and cardiovascular disease.

Best Natural Sources: Unrefined salts

There are three basic types of salt: standard table salt, sea salt and rock salt. Within these three categories there are several different salts each with a differing source and chemical make-up.

The Good: Unrefined salts are generally best as they contain a broad spectrum of trace elements. Unrefined salts may be either mined from the earth or harvested from the sea. These include rock salt and sea salt, but be sure that they are unrefined.

Types include Murray River Salt harvested from the rich red earth soil of the Murray Darling Basin region in Australia; Maldon Salt made from sea water drawn from the river Blackwater in Essex; Cornish Sea Salt harvested from water drawn straight out of the ocean off the Cornish coast; Welsh Halen Môn made from water drawn from the Menai Straits; Celtic sea salt (also known as Fleur de sel) harvested off the shores of Brittany; Himalayan salt (also known as Halite or Rock Salt) from Pakistan near the Himalayas; Alaea salt, an unrefined Hawaiian sea salt.

Dead Sea salt is salt extracted or taken from the Dead Sea, which contains only 10% sodium chloride compared with 97% in sea water but it's generally only used for therapeutic purposes.

All of these salts will contribute to high blood pressure (which may lead to hypertension), however many taste better due to the presence of trace elements and so less is required to season your food.

The Bad and the Ugly: Refined salts have had all the trace elements removed leaving pure sodium chloride, often coupled with an anti-caking agent and sometimes added iodine.

Refined salt is usually sold as table salt. Pickling salt is also refined but has no anti-caking agents.

SUGAR (also see Carbohydate)

Sugar is a form of crystallised carbohydrate that has been highly refined, mainly into sucrose, lactose and fructose.

Toxicity Risk:

If fat toxicity or type 2 diabetes is present then glucose toxicity is likely to follow where excess sugar binds proteins, which in turn produces advanced glycosolated end-products, or waste products that the body cannot get rid of, leading to premature ageing, impotence and eye, heart and kidney disease.

The Good:

No sugar is good, but the best replacement is pure Stevia – it's been used for 1,500 years by the Guaraní people of South America and it doesn't cause a spike in blood sugar levels.

Stevia is extracted from the leaves of the plant species Stevia rebaudiana, it's 150 times as sweet as sugar and often has an unpleasant metallic aftertaste. Keep in mind that of the Stevia sold is not 'pure' but highly processed, often chemically processed and bleached.

Monk fruit (siraitia grosvenorii or luo han guo) is nearly 300 times as sweet as sugar and has been dried, ground and used by Chinese monks since the 1200's. Whilst it's almost no calories and doesn't spike your blood sugar, commercially available monk fruit is highly processed and chemically treated to remove a number of 'interesting' sulphur-like flavours.

Erythritol is a sugar alcohol 60-70% as sweet as sucrose, but with almost no calories. It's often combined with Stevia to reduce the 'metallic' flavour, such as in SteviaSlim™.

Xylitol (a sugar alcohol with a low GI of 7) doesn't spike blood sugar either, but it is toxic to pets (especially dogs) causing often fatal hypoglycaemia.

Apart from pure Stevia, use of these 'artificial' sugar alcohols is preferable to other refined sugars due to their low calories and low GI.

The Bad:

Fruit pulp is the next best option because it causes a lower blood sugar spike, mostly because of the fibre that accompanies its fructose and glucose.

High sugar fruits, like dates, mangoes, watermelon, pineapple, banana, kiwi and grapes should be used in moderation in recipes.

And the Ugly: All other sugars including barley malt, rice bran syrup, blackstrap molasses, demerara, muscovado, honey, dates, pure maple syrup, palm sugar, coconut sugar, fruit juice concentrates, regular corn syrup, sucanat (granulated cane juice), refined crystalised sugars (white, brown, cane, beet), high fructose corn syrup, agave syrup, invert sugar syrup and anything with "ose" on the end should be avoided as much as possible, Marketing attempts may try to convince you they are acceptable sugars, but they're not.

Sugar is a highly addictive substance that is not easy to give up. Withdrawal symptoms include headaches, mood swings, depression, fatigue, and cravings. Sugar is such a huge weakness for me that I try to eliminate it. If I do start to eat sugar I want more and more until I am so overloaded that I end up falling asleep.

It is one of the most difficult substances to give up, not just because of its addictive nature, but because it's so prevalent and is hidden in many processed foods both savoury and sweet. This is one of the main reasons it's so important to avoid processed and fast foods – you just don't know it's in there.

Sugar has long had a link with type 2 diabetes, but it's also well known for its contributions to heart disease, osteoporosis, kidney disease, liver disease, obesity, depression and cancer. But did you know that a tablespoon of sugar can depresses the immune system for up to six hours? It also encourages candida, yeast infections, digestive problems and asthma.

When a friend of mine was diagnosed with cancer part of his treatment program included giving up all sugars due to their cancer causing links. Google "sugar" and you'll find that it's a major factor in a lot of degenerative diseases. We all know that too much sugar is bad, but even a little has far reaching consequences of which we may not be aware.

Types of sugars include the ordinary supermarket varieties (white, brown, raw, icing, caster) but high fructose corn syrup is one of the most common sugar ingredients in medicines and processed foods, many of which are labelled as being good for you.

Unfortunately the sugar and corn companies are so powerful at lobbying the Governments that we are unlikely to see a reduction in the use of corn syrup as an additive. So it's critical that you read all your food labels very carefully. Basically any word that ends in 'ose' is a sugar – glucose, sucrose, fructose, maltose, lactose, dextrose, galactose, and so on. Also avoid foods that contain other names for sugar like monosaccharides, disaccharides, syrups, sucanat, turbinado, demerara, muscovado, or evaporated cane juice.

Sugar Substitutes

If, like me, you like the taste of food with sugar (or have a sweet tooth) then there are some options that give you the taste of sugar.

The best option is SteviaSlim™ which a blend of Stevia and Erythritol. It's twice as sweet as sugar but has almost zero calories.

The other option is Xylitol. It might taste like sugar but beware - it's deadly to many pets, especially dogs.

The last option is to get used to the taste of Stevia, or better still retrain your palate and use no sugar at all!

Sugar substitutes like Splenda and Equal are artificially made and not really okay to use, even in very small quantities, simply because we don't really know the long term effects of these artificial sweeteners on the human body. And as this eating plan is all about only putting natural foods in your body you have to ask yourself whether consuming these is a wise option.

Refer to the following table for details of common sugar supplements.

Name	About	Safety / Side Effects
Agave Syrup	• Processed plant-based sweetener • Low GI comparable to fructose • Sweeter than honey and about 1.6 times as sweet as sugar • Less calories than sugar • Often used as a honey replacement for vegans	• Safe but consume in moderation
Aspartame	• Chemical creation • Odourless, white crystalline powder • Amino acid based (aspartic acid and phenylalanine.) • 200 times as sweet as sugar • Not suitable for cooking • Bitter aftertaste	• Reportedly safe in small quantities except for people with the genetic condition phenylketonuria
Cyclamate	• Artificial Chemical • 30-50 times as sweet as sugar • Bitter aftertaste and commonly combined with Saccharin • Still used in Europe but Banned in US	• Approved for use in over 100 countries • In US originally considered safe in 1958 but subsequently banned by FDA in 1969
Mannitol	• Polyol (sugar alcohol) • 50% as sweet as sucrose • Low calorie • Does not stimulate an increase in blood glucose • Often used in diabetic foods and medicines	• Reportedly safe except for patients with anuria or congestive heart failure • Doses larger than 20g can cause laxative effects
Melitose	Refer to Raffinose	
Neotame	• Artificial sweetener made by NutraSweet • 7,000 to 13,000 times sweeter than sugar • Has more of an aftertaste than sucralose	• Reportedly safe, approved by FDA in 2002

Name	About	Safety / Side Effects
PureVia	• Sold in USA • Developed by PepsiCo & Merisant • Contains dextrose, cellulose powder, natural flavors as well as the stevia extract rebaudioside A • As sweet as sugar • 90% less calories than sugar	• Reportedly safe, FDA approved December 2008 • This is a relatively new product with little consumption history
Raffinose	• Natural trisaccharide composed of galactose, fructose, and glucose found in vegetables (like asparagus, beans, cabbage and brussel sprouts) and whole grains • 30% as sweet as sugar	• Reportedly safe • Can cause flatulence
Saccharin	• Artificial chemical sweetener • 300 to 500 times as sweet as sugar • Zero calories • Often used to improve the taste of toothpastes, dietary foods, and dietary beverages. • Bitter or metallic aftertaste • Commonly sold as Sweet'n'Low in the US	• Reportedly safe in small quantities • Commercialised in early 1900's and became popular with the 60's and 70's diet crazes.
Sorbitol	• Naturally occurring sugar alcohol found in apples, pears, prunes and many stone fruit • Often used in toothpastes • 35% less calories than sugar • In digestion converts to fructose	• Reportedly safe • Can have a laxative effect
Splenda	Refer to Sucralose	

Name	About	Safety / Side Effects
Stevia	• Natural Sweetener / Herbal supplement • 300 times as sweet as sugar • Sold in health food stores • Banned in USA (not approved by FDA due to lobbying) • Taste is sweet but doesn't taste like sugar • Aftertaste can be like licorice in high concentrations	• No reported side effects • Considered safe • Used for more than 1500 years in South America • First cultivated in Japan for commercial use in 1971
Sucralose	• Artificial sweetener • Chlorinated sugar prepared from either sucrose or raffinose • 600 times as sweet as sugar • Stable under heat • Generally mixed with fillers, like maltodextrin and/or dextrose to produce a 1:1 by volume replacement for sugar • Pure sucralose has no calories but the fillers do	• Reportedly safe • First approved for use in Canada in 1991
SucraPlus	Refer to Sucralose	
Sucaryl	Refer to Cyclamate	
Sukrana	Refer to Sucralose	
Truvia	• Sugar substitute made of stevia extract rebiana, erythritol, and natural flavors • Developed by Coca-Cola & Cargill and is now #2 sugar substitute in USA • 2-3 times as sweet as sugar	• Reportedly safe, FDA approved December 2008 • This is a relatively new product with little consumption history

Name	About	Safety / Side Effects
Xylitol	• Naturally occurring sugar alcohol in the fibers of many fruits and vegetables • Same sweetness as sugar • Only two-thirds the calories	• Safe in regular amounts • Excess consumption can cause bloating, flatulence and diarrhoea • Very dangerous for dogs (due to differing metabolism from humans)

New Additions

Name	About	Safety / Side Effects
Coconut Sugar	• Also known as Coconut Palm Sugar • Made from the sap of the coconut palm with is then evaporated • Consists of up to 45% fructose / 55% sucrose • Lower GI (35) than regular sugar (60 to 75) • Contains more nutrients, vitamins and minerals than other sugars, and inulin which slows sugar absorption and helps boost immunity and gut health	• Should be treated the same way as sugar and avoided • No side effects other than those for any other sugar • High in calories • Spikes blood sugar just like regular sugar • Marketing hype is completely false and unfounded. It is not a 'super food' or healthy sugar option.
Erythritol	• Natural sugar alcohol made by fermentating corn, then crystalising the liquid • 60-70% as sweet as sucrose • Almost zero calories • Does not spike blood sugar • No tooth decay	• Second safest sweetener next to pure Stevia • In large doses (over 50g or 1.7 oz) can cause minor side effects of diarrhoea, stomach upset, and headache

Name	About	Safety / Side Effects
Monk Fruit	• Naturally dried and ground version has been used by Chinese monks since 1200's • Almost zero calories • Does not spike blood sugar	• Can cause allergic reactions in people who have gourd allergies. • No other known side effects • Purportedly has anti-inflammatory and anti-microbial properties • Commercial production is highly processed and highly chemically treated to remove unpleasant smells
Rice Bran Syrup	• Also known as Rice Malt Syrup or Brown Rice Syrup • Made from brown rice by breaking down its starches into 3 glucose modelecules • Contains 52% Maltotriose, 45% maltose and 3% glucose	• Should be treated the same way as sugar and avoided • No side effects other than those for any other sugar • High GI of 98 • High in calories (more than table sugar by volume) • No nutritional value • Spikes blood sugar just like regular sugar
SteviaSlim™	• Blend of Stevia and Erythritol • 2 to 3 times as sweet as sugar	• Refer individual ingredients

VITAMINS, MINERALS & TRACE ELEMENTS

Vitamins are either water soluble or fat soluble. Water-soluble vitamins don't store well in the body and tend to get depleted fast with deficiency occurring in a relatively short time. As a result the body needs a regular intake of these, preferably from natural sources, but you can use supplements if your dietary intake is insufficient.

Fat soluble vitamins are taken into the body via the digestion of fat and because they are not water soluble they store well (in adipose tissue and organs) and do not deplete easily. The body requires the correct levels of fat in order to absorb these vitamins, as well as the correct levels of water-soluble vitamins in order to metabolise fat. All very yin yang.

Let's now take a quick look at each vitamin, mineral and trace element required by the body.

◆◆

Ascorbic Acid:	See Vitamin C (also known as L-ascorbic acid)

◆◆

Beta-carotene:	Vitamin
Importance:	As a precursor of Vitamin A and a powerful antioxidant.
Deficiency Diseases:	A low dietary intake of carotenoids such as beta-carotene is not known to directly

cause any diseases or health conditions; however beta-carotene assists greatly with Vitamin A uptake and minimises damage from free radicals

RDI Adult:	700 – 3,000 micrograms
Toxicity Risk:	Rare but over consumption > 60 milligrams can lead to an enlarged liver; low blood pressure; orange colouration of the skin.
Best Natural Sources:	Green leafy and red and orange vegetables and fruits including asparagus, broccoli, Brussels sprouts, carrots, green beans, peas, red capsicum, spinach, sweet potato, tomato, winter squash, apricots, cantaloupe, orange, peaches, watermelon.

◆◆◆

Bioflavonoids:	Vitamin
Importance:	As a powerful antioxidant and immune system supporter; also known as flavonoids.
Deficiency Diseases:	Bruising easily; injuries and wounds not healing quickly.
RDI Adult:	30 – 3,000 milligrams
Toxicity Risk:	Non-toxic to humans however high doses may lead to diarrhoea
Best Natural Sources:	Broccoli, onion, tomato, apple, cranberry, strawberry, black tea and red wine.

❖ ❖

Biotin: See Vitamin H

❖ ❖

Boron: Mineral

Importance: Helps prevent bone loss and demineralisation.

Deficiency Diseases: Osteoporosis, decreased blood levels of oestrogen and testosterone.

RDI Adult: 2 – 20 milligrams

Toxicity Risk: Highly toxic if taken in high doses, leading to headache; nausea; vomiting; diarrhoea; kidney damage; hair loss and doses approaching18 grams (0.6 oz) can lead to circulatory collapse and death.

Buddies: Calcium and Magnesium

Best Natural Sources: Avocado, broccoli, carrot, celery, apple, dried apricot, dates, prunes, raisins, almond, brazil nut, cashew, hazelnut, walnut, red kidney beans, lentils, olives and red wine.

❖ ❖

Calcium: Mineral

Importance: Metallic element for neurotransmitter release, muscle contraction including heart function. 99% of the body's calcium is stored in bones and teeth.

Deficiency Diseases:	Osteoporosis; rickets; poor blood clotting; impaired kidney function; decreased absorption of other minerals.
RDI Adult:	1,000 – 2,500 milligrams
Toxicity Risk:	Low, but doses in excess of 1.4 grams per kilogram of body weight can lead to asthma; memory problems; muscle weakness; and depression. Excessive consumption of calcium carbonate antacids over a period of weeks or months can cause issues including renal failure. People taking some medications, or with kidney disease, should not take supplements.
Buddies:	Boron, Vitamin D and Magnesium
Best Natural Sources:	Beans, broccoli, cabbage, kale hijiki, kelp, okra, sweet potato, seaweed, wakame, figs, quinoa, almonds, peanuts, sesame, sunflower seeds, fish, milk and dairy products, fortified soy milk, powdered eggshell.

◆◆

Chloride:	Mineral
Importance:	Electrolyte that helps controls the flow of fluid in body tissue and blood vessels, and also regulates body acidity.
Deficiency Diseases:	Rare, but low levels may lead to excessive loss of potassium; weakness; and lowered blood pressure.
RDI Adult:	2,300 – 3,600 milligrams

Toxicity Risk:	None identified due to being water soluble, however high levels may lead to fluid retention.
Buddies:	Potassium and sodium
Best Natural Sources:	Celery, tomato, kelp, olives, table salt.

❖❖

Choline:	Vitamin
Importance:	Part of the B-complex group that helps brain and memory development, liver function, cell activity and nutrient transport.
Deficiency Diseases:	Fatty liver; kidney problems; high blood pressure; deterioration of memory and brain function.
RDI Adult:	425 – 3,500 milligrams
Toxicity Risk:	Doses in excess of 3.5 grams can lead to trimethylaminuria; kidney disease; liver disease; depression; and Parkinson's disease.
Buddy:	Inositol
Best Natural Sources:	Lecithin, beans, peas, spinach, eggs, fish, liver, muscle meats, bacon, nuts, and wheat germ although the body can make its own quantities of choline.

❖❖

Chromium:	Mineral
Importance:	Helps the body to maintain a stable blood glucose level by controlling insulin and some enzymes. Chromium picolinate is the best absorbed type of chromium but will only be absorbed as a supplement if the body has a deficiency.
Deficiency Diseases:	Low levels of chromium are very common and lead to anxiety; fatigue; glucose intolerance; and atherosclerosis.
RDI Adult:	25 – 35 micrograms
Toxicity Risk:	200 micrograms, and exposure to environmental chromium long-term may lead to skin, liver and kidney problems.
Best Natural Sources:	Broccoli, green beans, potato, orange, grapes, beef, turkey.

✦✦

Cobalt:	Mineral
Importance:	An essential B_{12} trace element necessary for healthy thyroid function. Aids in forming healthy red blood cells.
Deficiency Diseases:	Anaemia via a deficiency of B_{12}.
RDI Adult:	0.12 – 2 micrograms
Toxicity Risk:	Greater than 30 milligrams per day can lead to hot flushes; skin rashes; vomiting; nausea; diarrhoea; pneumonociosis; possible reduction in male fertility; and

inhibits iodine uptake which can further lead to goitre; and hypothyroidism.

Buddy: Vitamin B_{12}

Best Natural Sources: Mostly in seafood, fish, red meat, milk, and some in nuts and leafy green vegetables.

◆◆◆

Copper: Mineral

Importance: Antioxidant required for the formation of red blood cells, elastin, collagen, melanin and healthy bones.

Deficiency Diseases: Rare, as copper is stored in the body, however very low levels can lead to anaemia; osteoporosis; thyroid problems; heart and nervous system disease; and an increase in infection.

RDI Adult: 0.9 - 10 milligrams

Toxicity Risk: Doses exceeding 40 milligrams can lead to Wilson's disease; tachycardia; high blood pressure; coma; and death.

Buddy: Iron

Best Natural Sources: Mushroom, shellfish, liver, almonds, cashew, hazelnut, sunflower seed, lentils and chocolate.

◆◆◆

Cyanocobalamin: See Vitamin B_{12}

◆◆◆

Fluoride:	Mineral
Importance:	Helps prevent tooth decay; promotes strong teeth and bones.
Deficiency Diseases:	Rare, due to fluoridation of water supplies.
RDI Adult:	3 – 10 milligrams
Toxicity Risk:	Doses greater than 30 milligrams can lead to white spots on teeth; nausea; vomiting; diarrhoea; abdominal pain; and fluorosis.
Buddies:	Iron, Magnesium and Molybdenum
Best Natural Sources:	Tap water, asparagus, carrot, spinach, raisins, red wine.

◆◆◆

Folate / Folic Acid:	See Vitamin B

◆◆◆

Inositol:	Vitamin
Importance:	Part of the B-complex group that aids cell health in the brain, bone marrow, eyes and intestines, and also promotes healthy hair growth.
Deficiency Diseases:	Rarely occur, but low levels of inositol can lead to constipation; eczema; elevated cholesterol levels; and hair loss.
RDI Adult:	30 – 3,000 milligrams
Toxicity Risk:	Essentially non-toxic to humans, however high doses can lead to diarrhoea; and

increased secretion of creatine.

Buddy:	Choline
Best Natural Sources:	Vegetables, bananas, raisins, liver, nuts, oat flakes, brown rice, wheat germ and brewer's yeast.

❖❖❖

Iodine:	Mineral
Importance:	An essential trace element for thyroid function and regulation of basal metabolic rate.
Deficiency Diseases:	Hypothyroidism; possible breast and stomach cancer.
Toxicity Risk:	Doses greater than 1,500 micrograms can lead to decreased thyroid activity; stomach irritation; goitre; Grave's disease; hyperthyroidism; swollen heart; and hypersensitivity.
RDI Adult:	0.15 – 1.1 milligrams
Buddy:	Selenium
Best Natural Sources:	Kelp, iodised table salt, shellfish.

❖❖❖

Iron: Mineral

Deficiency Diseases: Anaemia; but low levels can also lead to
                            fatigue; memory issues; and poor
                            immunity.

Toxicity Risk: Doses in excess of 20 milligrams per
                            kilogram of body weight can lead to
                            metabolic acidosis; shock; liver
                            failure; coagulopathy; adult respiratory
                            distress syndrome; long-term organ
                            damage; and coma. Doses in excess of
                            60 milligrams per kilogram of body
                            weight, usually only achievable via use of
                            iron supplements, can lead to death.

RDI Adult: 8 - 18 milligrams

Buddy   Copper, increased absorption with
                            vitamin C and organic acids such as
                            citric, lactic or malic.

Best Natural Sources: Red meat, poultry, fish, beans, leaf
                            vegetables, lentils, tofu, chickpeas,
                            black-eyed peas.

••

Magnesium: Mineral

Importance: An enzyme catalyst essential for all cells
                            of all living organisms.

Deficiency Diseases: Asthma, diabetes and osteoporosis.

Toxicity Risk: Low due to excretion by kidney, unless over supplemented but doses in excess of 2,000 milligrams can lead to low blood pressure; muscle weakness; sleepiness; thirst; nausea; vomiting; paralysis of the central nervous system; difficulty breathing, and; irregular heartbeats.

RDI Adult:	310 - 420 milligrams
Buddy:	Boron
Best Natural Sources:	Vegetables (particularly green leafy), broccoli, peas, potato, spinach, banana, legumes, spices, almonds, cashews, peanuts, walnuts, tofu, milk, dairy products, cereals, coffee, cocoa, tea.

◆◆

Manganese:	Mineral
Importance:	Activates enzymes that aid with the metabolism of carbohydrates, amino acids and cholesterol, enables the body to use Vitamins C, B1, H and choline and helps prevent diabetes.
Deficiency Diseases:	Rare although low levels may lead to problems with glucose levels; poor bone growth; reduced fertility, and; birth defects.
RDI Adult:	1.8 – 11 milligrams
Toxicity Risk:	Doses greater than 50 milligrams can lead to anaemia; high blood pressure; insomnia; mental problems; kidney inflammation; tremors; muscle fatigue; anorexia, and; impotence.

Best Natural Sources:	Sweet potato, pineapple, almonds, peanuts, pecans, brown rice, navy beans, pinot beans, lima beans, green tea and black tea.

◆◆

Molybdenum:	Mineral
Importance:	Needed for normal cell function, nitrogen metabolism and fights nitrosamines associated with cancer.
Deficiency Diseases:	Never observed
RDI Adult:	45 – 2,000 micrograms
Toxicity Risk:	Doses greater than 2,000 micrograms can lead to diarrhoea; gout; and anaemia.
Best Natural Sources:	Dark leafy green vegetables, peas, spinach, liver, milk, lima beans and grains.

◆◆

Niacin:	See Vitamin B_3

◆◆

Pantothenic Acid:	See Vitamin B_5

◆◆

Para-Amino Benzoic Acid (PABA):	Vitamin
Importance:	Part of the B-complex group that helps improve protein use, red blood cell

formation and the manufacture of folic acid. PABA also helps to block ultraviolet rays and is an ingredient in sunscreens.

Deficiency Diseases:	None, although low doses may lead to fatigue; irritability; nervousness; depression; constipation; patchy, itchy areas on the skin; and weeping eczema.
RDI Adult:	10 – 1,000 milligrams
Toxicity Risk:	Not determined although high doses may lead to anorexia; fever; nausea; and rashes.
Buddies:	Folic Acid, Vitamin B5
Best Natural Sources:	Beans, green leafy vegetables, lentils, organ meats (liver, heart, kidney, etc) eggs and yeast.

◆◆◆

Phosphorus:	Mineral
Importance:	Plays a major role in the biological molecules of all living organisms, important for the effective utilization of B-group vitamins energy metabolism and the formation of bone and teeth.
Deficiency Diseases:	Rare, however cases of extreme insufficiency can lead to anaemia; muscle weakness; rickets; osteomalacia, and; hypophosphatemia.
RDI Adult:	700 – 4,000 milligrams
Toxicity Risk:	Doses exceeding 5,000 milligrams can lead

to bone re-absorption; calcification of heart and kidney; osteoporosis; hypocalcaemia, and; secondary parathyroidism. Some organic compounds of phosphorus are toxic, and over ingestion can lead to kidney damage and osteoporosis.

Buddies:	Helps with the body's ability to use iron, calcium, magnesium, and zinc.
Best Natural Sources:	Tuna, salmon, sardines and shellfish, liver, beef, chicken, turkey, milk and dairy products, eggs, almonds, brazil nut, cashew, pistachio, walnut, sesame seed, curry powder, pepper and cocoa powder.

◆◆◆

Potassium:	Mineral
Importance:	An electrolyte that maintains fluid balances, assists with muscle function and the transmission of nerve impulses as well as carbohydrate and protein metabolism.
Deficiency Diseases:	Hypokalaemia, hypertension and diarrhoea.
RDI Adult:	4,700 milligrams
Toxicity Risk:	Generally only when kidneys aren't functioning, however doses in excess of 10 grams (0.35 oz) can lead to dehydration; stomach upsets; intestinal problems; heart rhythm disorder; convulsions with extreme cases resulting in heart attack; and kidney failure.

Buddies:	Chloride and sodium
Best Natural Sources:	Avocado, broccoli, bamboo shoots, carrot, cauliflower, corn, parsley, potato, spinach, sweet potato, tomato, banana, kiwi fruit, orange, strawberries, dried apricot, almond, pistachio, soybeans, and bran, although all meats, vegetables and dairy all contain good sources.

◆◆◆

Riboflavin	See Vitamin B_2

◆◆◆

Selenium:	Mineral
Importance:	An essential micronutrient for thyroid function.
Deficiency Diseases:	Thyroid gland problems; Keshan's Disease; and Kashin-Beck Disease.
RDI Adult:	55 - 400 micrograms
Toxicity Risk:	Doses in excess of 1,000 micrograms can lead to fatigue, nausea, liver impairment; selenosis; and extreme cases may result in cirrhosis of the liver; pulmonary oedema; and death.
Best Natural Sources:	Mushrooms, brazil nut, black walnut, beef, chicken, kidney, tuna, crab, salmon, prawns, lobster, eggs, brown rice and milk.

◆◆◆

Silica: Mineral, also known as silicon dioxide

Importance: Trace element that promotes the health of bones, cartilage, tendons, blood vessels and artery walls.

Deficiency Diseases: Hardening of the arteries and decay of teeth and bones.

RDI Adult: 9 – 30 milligrams

Toxicity Risk: Doses over 700 milligrams may lead to kidney damage. People with oedema should avoid supplements.

Best Natural Sources: Mineral water, alfalfa, beetroot, carrot, green beans, lettuce, onions, banana, raisin, barley, brown rice, millet and oats.

◆ ◆

Sodium: Mineral

Importance: An electrolyte required by the body to keep fluid levels in balance, and combines to form hydrochloric acid in the stomach.

Deficiency Diseases: Only occurs if daily intake is less than 500mg, or in cases of severe vomiting and/ or diarrhoea.

RDI Adult: 0.9 – 2.3 grams (0.03 – 0.8 oz)

Toxicity Risk: Doses greater than 18 grams per day can lead to Diarrhoea; excessive salivation; excessive thirst; exhaustion; fluid retention; hyperactivity; seizures; tremors;

and high blood pressure.

Buddies: Potassium and chloride

Best Natural Sources: Sodium is used in high concentrations in most processed foods and is naturally present in carrot, tomato, mango, almond and brown rice.

◆◆

Thiamine: See Vitamin B_1, also known as Thiamin

◆◆

Tocopherol: See Vitamin E

◆◆

Vanadium: Mineral

Importance: Trace element that contributes to bone development and reproduction.

Deficiency Diseases: Elevation of LDL, reduced bone growth and reproduction.

RDI Adult: 0.5 – 1.8 milligrams

Toxicity Risk: Doses greater than 2.5 milligrams can lead to negative effects on the uptake of choline, vitamin C, chromium and magnesium.

Best Natural Sources: Mushroom, olives, shellfish, black pepper and vegetable oils.

◆◆

Vitamin A: Vitamin

Importance: Used by the retina of the eye and necessary
                                 for both low-light and colour vision and by
                                 the body for immune function, gene
                                 transportation, bone metabolism, skin and
                                 cellular health.

Deficiency Diseases: Sinusitis; skin disorders; dry skin and
                                 hair; frequent cold and respiratory infections;
                                 dryness of the eyes eventually leading to
                                 night blindness and possible blindness.

RDI Adult: 700 – 3,000 micrograms

Toxicity Risk: Hypervitaminosis A but only from high
                                 supplement intake.

Buddy: Vitamin A is fat-soluble and needs fat in
                                 the diet for uptake.

Best Natural Sources: Broccoli, carrot, collard greens, dandelion
                                 greens, kale, pea, pumpkin, spinach,
                                 sweet potato, cantaloupe, apricot, papaya,
                                 mango, meat (liver, beef, pork, chicken,
                                 turkey, fish especially swordfish and
                                 salmon), cheddar cheese, milk, butter, egg
                                 and cod liver oil.

◆◆

Vitamin B: Vitamin

Importance: Naturally occurs as folate and is particularly
                                 important for children and pregnant
                                 women as it's important for synthesizing
                                 and repairing DNA, cell division and
                                 growth, and preventing anaemia.

Deficiency Diseases: Pregnancy complications and poor development of embryos; impaired DNA synthesis and repair possibly leading to cancer.

RDI Adult: 400 – 1,000 micrograms

Buddy: Vitamin B_{12}

Toxicity Risk: Low, however due to being water soluble daily doses in excess of 7,150 micrograms can lead to abdominal bloating; flatulence; hyperactivity; irritability; nausea, and; and sleep disturbances. Folic acid prevents epilepsy and anti-convulsive medications from working properly.

Best Natural Sources: Avocado, asparagus, beans, beets, broccoli, Brussels sprouts, corn, peas, spinach, banana, cantaloupe, orange, lentils, chickpeas, lima beans, kidney beans, liver, kidney, egg yolk, sunflower seeds and peanut.

◆◆

Vitamin B_1: Vitamin

Importance: An enzyme assister to enable carbohydrate to be used as energy. Also important for brain, nerve and heart function.

Deficiency Diseases: Rare however the nervous system and the heart are particularly sensitive to thiamine deficiency and low doses can lead to severe fatigue of eyes and myriad problems including Neurodegeneration; Beriberi, and; Wernicke-Korsakoff syndrome. Also deficiency prevents ability to use glucose normally and may cause complications for diabetics and those with hypoglycaemia.

RDI Adult:

0.7 – 1.4 milligrams

Toxicity Risk:

Rare however daily doses over 125 milligrams per kilogram of body weight can lead to tachycardia; shortness of breath; sweating; tremors; hot flushes; nervousness; and fluid retention.

Best Natural Sources:

Asparagus, cauliflower, corn, kale, peas, potatoes, oranges, meat (liver, beef, pork, and chicken), oatmeal, flax, cashew, pecans, sunflower seeds, brown rice, whole grain rye, eggs, yeast and yeast extract. Destroyed by alcohol and tea tannins so drink them well after a meal.

◆◆

Vitamin B$_2$:

Vitamin

Importance:

Assists a variety of cellular processes and plays a key role in the metabolism of fats, ketone bodies, carbohydrates and proteins. Note that exposure to light destroys riboflavin.

Deficiency Diseases:

Rare, however symptoms of low doses such as scaly skin; red eyes; and anaemia may present but levels in humans don't usually get to the point where disease occurs.

RDI Adult: 1.1 – 1.3 milligrams

Toxicity Risk: Essentially not-toxic to humans if taken orally.

Best Natural Sources: Asparagus, chard, green bean, mushroom, okra, tomato, leafy green vegetables, sweet potato, banana, persimmon, legumes, cheese, cottage cheese, milk, yogurt, meat, kidneys, liver, egg, salmon, almond and yeast.

• •

Vitamin B$_3$:   Vitamin

Importance: Blocks the breakdown of special fats to decrease the secretion of VLDL and cholesterol by the liver thereby increasing the amount of HDL or good cholesterol in the body.

Deficiency Diseases: Rare, however symptoms of low doses such as scaly skin, red eyes, and anaemia may present. Extreme deficiencies may lead to Pellagra, hereditary Hartnup's disease and some psychiatric issues.

RDI Adult: 14 – 35 milligrams

Toxicity Risk: Rare, but daily doses exceeding 1.4 grams per kilogram of body weight may lead to flushing; burning or itchy skin; diarrhoea; increased heart and breathing rates; high blood pressure; and liver abnormalities.

Best Natural Sources:	Asparagus, avocado, broccoli, carrots, leaf vegetables, mushroom, sweet potato, tomato, nectarine, beef, chicken, fish, salmon, tuna, heart, kidney, liver, milk, cottage cheese, egg, peanut, brown and wild rice, cereal, legumes and brewer's yeast (e.g. Vegemite).

◆◆◆

Vitamin B_5:	Vitamin
Importance:	Assists co-enzyme manufacture that assists the conversion of fats and carbohydrates into energy; assists with hormone, red blood cell and Vitamin D production.
Deficiency Diseases:	None, long term alcoholics may tend toward low levels of all B-group vitamins.
RDI Adult:	5 milligrams
Toxicity Risk:	Essentially non-toxic to humans although doses in excess of 10 grams (0.35 oz) may lead to diarrhoea.
Buddies:	Vitamin B_1, B_2, B_3, B_6 and Vitamin H
Best Natural Sources:	Broccoli, corn, mushrooms, potato, sweet potato, tomato, liver, meat (fresh not frozen), milk, yoghurt, egg, wheat germ, oats, chick peas, lentils, lima beans.

◆◆

Vitamin B$_6$:   Vitamin

Importance: Helps convert stored carbohydrates into a usable form, ingested proteins into usable proteins, and is a co-enzyme to many other enzymes in the body that are involved predominantly in metabolism.

Deficiency Diseases: Anaemia; low levels can compromise the immune system, leading to dermatologic and neurologic changes and a predisposition to ill health.

RDI Adult: 1.3 to 100 milligrams

Toxicity Risk: Low, due to being water soluble. However daily doses above 100 milligrams can lead to pain and numbness of the extremities and difficulty walking.

Best Natural Sources: Avocado, Brussels sprouts, cabbage, carrots, corn, green capsicum, parsley, potato, sweet potato, apple, avocado, banana, dried apricots, raisins, sultanas, dates, prunes, hazelnut, walnut, liver, beef, chicken, pork, veal, milk and dairy products and whole grain products. The cooking, freezing, canning, storage and processing of foods can lead to losses of up to 50% of vitamin B$_6$ so fresh is best.

$\bullet$

Vitamin B$_{12}$:   Vitamin

Importance: Assists in normal functioning of the brain and nervous system, and for the formation of blood.

Deficiency Diseases: Low levels can cause irreversible damage to the brain and nervous system, as well as anaemia.

RDI Adult: 2 - 3 micrograms per day

Toxicity Risk: Essentially non-toxic to humans due to being water soluble.

Buddies: all Vitamin B group and Calcium

Best Natural Sources: Foods that come from animals including fish and shellfish, meat (especially liver), poultry, eggs, milk, and milk products. Vegans should eat fortified soy products and/or take a dietary supplement.

◆◆

Vitamin C: Vitamin

Importance: An antioxidant and essential nutrient used for metabolic reactions and to lessen oxidative stress, natural antihistamine, immune system support and used to make collagen.

Deficiency Diseases: Scurvy. Vitamin C is depleted by the consumption of antacids, alcohol, anti-depressants and birth control pills.

RDI Adult: 75 – 2,000 milligrams

Toxicity Risk:	Low, due to being water soluble. However large doses may cause indigestion and diarrhoea and will also increase iron absorption placing people with the genetic disease haemochromatosis at risk of iron poisoning.

Buddy: Bioflavonoids

Best Natural Sources:	All fruits and green vegetables, particularly broccoli, Brussels sprouts, green chilli pepper, parsley, red pepper, wild potato, camu camu fruit, goji berry, kakadu plum, kiwi fruit, loganberry, lychee, persimmon, redcurrant, rose hip. Citrus fruits (orange, lemons, limes, etc) have less vitamin C but are still valuable sources, as are papaya, strawberry and garlic. Vitamin C can be lost from food when it's cooked.

◆◆◆

Vitamin D:	Vitamin
Importance:	Helps to regulate the absorption of calcium and supports the immune system.
Deficiency Diseases:	Rickets; osteomalacia
RDI Adult:	5 – 50 micrograms
Toxicity Risk:	Dosages exceeding 50 micrograms per day (usually from supplements) can cause calcium deposits in soft tissues of the body including the blood vessel walls and kidneys where it can cause serious damage.

Buddies:	Boron, Magnesium, Vitamin B5 and natural direct sunlight to the face – depending on the strength of the ultra violet light get 10 to 30 minutes per day for your body to produce the optimum amount of Vitamin D.
Best Natural Sources:	Cod liver oil, herring, mackerel, prawns, salmon, sardines, beef liver, milk and milk products and eggs.

◆◆

Vitamin E:	Vitamin
Importance:	A lipid-soluble antioxidant that has a regulatory effect on enzymatic activities.
Deficiency Diseases:	Spinocerebellar ataxia; myopathies; peripheral neuropathy; ataxia; skeletal myopathy; retinopathy; and impairment of the immune response.
RDI Adult:	15 – 1,000 milligrams
Toxicity Risk:	None, but daily intake greater than 2,000 milligrams can block vitamin A absorption and may induce diarrhoea, nausea or abdominal wind.
Best Natural Sources:	Leafy green vegetables (beets, collard, lettuce, spinach, turnip), asparagus, broccoli, pumpkin, sweet potato, tomato, avocado, mango, papaya, almond, hazelnut, wheat germ oil, sunflower oil, nut oils, blue crab, rockfish and olives.

• •

Vitamin H: Vitamin

Importance: Part of the B-complex group used to assist cell growth and the metabolism of fats and proteins.

Deficiency Diseases: Rare, but low levels can lead to hair thinning; depression; fatigue; dry scaly skin; and elevation of cholesterol levels.

RDI Adult: 30 milligrams

Toxicity Risk: None due to being water soluble

Best Natural Sources: Cauliflower, mushrooms, spinach, beef liver, chicken breast, salmon, nuts, cheese, eggs, brewer's yeast and can also be manufactured in the body should a small shortfall occur. Consumption of raw eggs, which contain avadin, can cause vitamin deficiency due to adavin's ability to bind with Vitamins B and H preventing uptake by the body.

• •

Vitamin K: Vitamin

Importance: Helps blood clot and prevents excess bleeding.

Deficiency Diseases: Rare, usually caused as a result of liver disease or a problem digesting fat. Slow blood clotting and nose bleeds are good indicators of low vitamin K levels.

Vitamin K also helps with calcium uptake to prevent osteoporosis.

RDI Adult:

30 micrograms

Toxicity Risk:

None, except over consumption greater than 100 micrograms of synthetic compound Menadione.

Buddy:

Dietary fat

Best Natural Sources:

Green leafy vegetables, broccoli, cabbage, carrots, cauliflower, green beans, parsley, peas, spinach, tomato, turnips, beef liver, milk, egg, soybean oil and fermented soy products.

◆◆

Zinc:

Mineral

Importance:

Vital to the immune system, keeps skin healthy and preserves eyesight.

Deficiency Diseases:

Rare, but low levels can lead to more frequent infections; skin irritations; slow wound healing; poor sense of taste; increased hair loss; male infertility; and/or prostate problems.

RDI Adult:

8 – 40 milligrams

Toxicity Risk:

Doses over 150 milligrams can lead to anaemia; lethargy; nausea; vomiting; increased LDL cholesterol; lowered HDL cholesterol; and dysfunction of the central nervous system.

Best Natural Sources:	Liver, beef, chicken, turkey, oysters, flounder, chickpeas, lentils, split peas, white beans, milk and dairy products, almond, cashew, peanut, sunflower seeds, walnut and egg.

•••

Okay, that's the long technical bit over. I know, it was a hard slog. So now that you've read it how do you implement it? How do make sure that your body is getting all the right nutrients in the correct quantities?

Did you notice most of the vitamins, minerals and trace elements have the same or similar best natural sources? Fresh fruit, vegetables, legumes, nuts, eggs, low fat dairy, some grains, fish and lean meats are the best sources because they obtain their nutrients (vitamins) from the soil or, in the case of eggs, dairy, fish and meat, are produced as a result of eating nutrient rich foods.

You don't see a Cadbury™ Creme Egg or Griffin's™ Toffee Pops biscuit in the list anywhere do you? No, and that's because they have little or no nutritional value. And this is also why most nutritionists recommend a diet high in fresh fruit and vegetables and low in packaged and processed foods.

And if you eat natural rather than processed foods, it is unlikely you will have to worry about taking vitamin and mineral supplements as you'll get all the nutrients you'll need. You also won't run the risk of accidentally overdosing on vitamin or mineral supplements.

Sounds simple, right? So if it's so simple, why doesn't everyone do it?

Is Organic Better?

There is little doubt that much of our farmed land is over farmed and artificially fertilised to produce quick large crops. Modern agricultural methods lead to nutrient depleted and chemically infused foods that are much less nutrient filled that those grown in rich organic soils.

As a result organic and biodynamic foods are better food sources, however, we can't all eat organic foods. Despite this type of produce becoming more readily available it is often expensive and much of it is uncertified. It is said there is $50 million worth of organic produce grown annually, but over $100 million sold.

Whilst organic and biodynamic is best, it's not critical. Don't get completely hung up about it. Swapping processed and packaged foods for fresh conventionally farmed produce will yield far greater results.

Do Supplements Work?

There are an abundance of weight loss supplements on the market today, many with unfounded claims as the new super cure for the obesity epidemic that society faces. Everything from diet and protein shakes, to mangosteen, metabolism boosters and everything in between. Many of us cling to these supplements in the hope they will make the difference, give us the edge, and be the panacea to the excess weight that has been plaguing us for so long – the solution to all our dreams and wishes.

It's time to face reality ~ most of these so called "supplements" don't work, at least not in the long term, or not without following a sensible diet and exercise plan, which would have yielded similar results even if you didn't take the supplement in the first place.

The weight loss industry creates a great deal of hype with respect to weight loss supplements almost solely to sell more products. According to the Mayo Clinic's research into weight loss supplements, very few actually work and many are considered unsafe. Most have 'reported' success when combined with dietary control and exercise (what a surprise), but little evidence exists to prove the supplements contributed any additional benefit to those derived from the dietary control and exercise itself.

> *"Weight loss supplements are generally not useful and have no place in a long-term nutritionally balanced diet."*

Weight loss supplements are generally not useful and have no place in a long-term nutritionally balanced diet. In many cases the money you spend on weight loss supplements would be better spent on whole foods or elsewhere in your life to help reach your goals.

If you are changing your diet to include an increase in fresh fruit and vegetables and lean meats you are less likely to need to take any supplements at all. However if your diet is lacking in some area, vitamin supplements (as opposed to weight loss supplements) may be useful and can play a major role in topping up your daily intake.

You might like to consider the following vitamin and herbal supplements that I have found useful in my journey.

VITAMINS

Multivitamins:

Multivitamins only contain a partial amount of your required dietary intake. They are designed to be an adjunct or top up to your normal food. But not all multivitamin preparations (or vitamin preparations for that matter) are equal. Most claim to have the best ingredients, or be the best for you, but many of them are driven by bottom line costs and maximum profits which means they contain cheap often synthetic ingredients, fillers and additives.

When choosing a multivitamin, you need to also consider how they are manufactured – up to 80% are contaminated or contain toxins, which is not what you, the consumer, signed up for in purchasing the product. Where possible you should only buy supplements produced in Good Manufacturing Practice (or GMP) certified or compliant facilities which have very rigorous manufacturing standards, similar to those required by law to produce pharmaceutical drugs.

And when you do find the right one, taking one vitamin supplement without another may not be at all beneficial to your body. This is because many vitamins require the presence of other vitamins for uptake into the body. This is why 'complete' or 'balanced' multi-vitamins have become so popular. Another thing to remember is that women and men can have quite different dietary requirements and therefore require a different balance of vitamins and minerals for optimal health.

Iodine:

If the thyroid gland controls your metabolism, then iodine is the throttle it uses. If your iodine tank is empty then your thyroid will be sluggish. And, metabolism slows as we grow older so if you're continually tired, irritable, depressed and having difficulty losing weight despite a good diet and lots of exercise, then an iodine supplement may be the answer for you.

How much iodine you need will depend on how deficient your body is. Fluoride, found in our water supplies and toothpastes actually leeches iodine from the body. There are over two dozen symptoms of iodine deficiency, including weight gain, low energy, brain fog, insomnia, ice-cold hands or feet, dry skin, hair loss, muscle pain, swollen ankles and elevated cholesterol.

Thyroid function tests may show your thyroid is operating within normal range, however your thyroid could be functioning at only 30% of peak efficiency, but your tests will say that's fine. I suggest getting tested to know your current iodine level, taking an iodine supplement for four or six weeks and then testing your levels again. If you're not closer to the higher end of the test range then, depending how you feel, you can increase your iodine supplement.

Fish Oil:

Research has shown that 1-2 grams (0.035 – 0.07 oz) of omega rich fish oil can help reduce sugar cravings and curb the appetite leading to greater weight loss results.

But fish oils provide many more benefits. It's the EPA and DHA in fish oil and fish oil supplements that contain extremely important omega 3 fatty acids being used to help prevent and treat many diseases. Fish oils also help prevent heart disease, high blood pressure, high cholesterol, inflammation and arthritis. Studies show it can also lower the risk of breast cancer in women.

L-Carnitine:

L-Carnitine is an amino acid, naturally produced by the body that acts to help transport fatty acids, delivering them into the mitochondria where they'll be oxidised and eventually converted into energy the body can use. However some people don't produce enough L-Carnitine and can benefit from a supplement. Be aware that L-Carnitine is not a cure all solution, it is an expensive aid to weight loss and requires a significant amount of exercise to be performed in order to gain results.

Only use L-Carnitine if you are having trouble shedding those last few kilograms and are performing a significant amount of cardio and resistance training.

HERBAL SUPPLEMENTS

Some herbal supplements can aid weight loss, usually by adding bulk to the diet, increasing metabolism, fat burning or nutritional intake, or enhancing one's mood.

Here are some of the more commonly used herbs, but remember that none of these herbal supplements have conclusive studies to support their claims and so caution should be used if relying on any of these to assist in your weight loss goals.

Bitter Orange	Inconclusive metabolism booster and may assist body fat loss. Caution for those with heart disease or high blood pressure.
Cayenne	Reputed to aid weight loss based on the principle that spices speed up your metabolism.
Hoodia gordonii	Supposed appetite suppressant where the steroidal glycoside P57 is present; also enhances weight loss by lowering blood glucose. Not shown to have significant side effects.
Coleus	Suspected to assist weight loss by breaking down fat deposits and preventing production of adipose tissue; mildly stimulates the metabolism by increasing thyroid function.
Ephedra	Clinical trials have shown benefit in weight loss but there are major safety concerns with this herb.
Green Tea	Purported metabolism booster via caffeine and a rich source of antioxidants, which is claimed aids weight loss.
Guarana	Reported metabolism booster because of its caffeine content.
Guggul	Possible metabolism booster and reducer of cholesterol levels.
Guar gum	A plant based dietary fibre derived from the bean of the plant.

Garcina Cambogia	Potential appetite suppressant and may reduce the body's ability to form adipose (fatty) tissue caused by overeating, by inhibiting the body's ability to convert carbohydrates to fats. Not recommended for pregnancy, diabetes, dementia syndromes or some prescription medicines.
Yerba Mate	Purported metabolism booster.
Spirulina	High value nutrient purported to satisfy hunger.
St. John's Wort	Mood enhancer, indirect assistance. Interferes with the contraceptive pill.

I personally haven't used all of these herbal supplements, however I do drink Green Tea on occasion and sometimes use either St John's Wort or Rhodiola (see *Get Your Body Right: Survive Stress*) daily among other herbal and vitamin supplements.

Water Works

The body excretes about 100 millilitres per hour, which equates to about two and a half litres of water per day. Whilst we do get some hydration from high water content vegetables, it is vital that we replace the lost water with pure water each and every day. This means we need to consume a minimum of 2.4 litres of pure water just to replace the fluids we lose each day.

Many of the drinks we consume actually dehydrate us further – coffee, tea, soft drinks and alcohol all tend to leave our body more dehydrated and they don't contribute at all to our water intake, in fact for every glass of non-water that we consume we need to consume an equal quantity of water on top of the minimum daily requirement. This is the reason that drinking water, as opposed to sports drinks, which contain artificial flavours, colours and unwanted sugars and salts (hidden behind words such as electrolytes), is much more beneficial for your body.

So the majority of people are actually chronically dehydrated. This can not only cause a myriad of ailments in the body, but also restrict brain function. For the body to function optimally the fluid balance is important, and in order to remove the waste products from weight loss the body's water supply is vital.

There are some schools of thought that believe you should be drinking 45ml per kilogram of body weight (or 3.4 fluid ounces to every pound of body weight), plus more if you're exercising, plus even more to offset the effects of drinks like caffeine that dehydrate.

For many years I believed this and regularly drank 4 litres (135.3 fluid ounces) each day. And for many years I was alright until in 2018 I was referred to an Endocrinologist because I was having some minor health issues. What transpired as I dropped off my 6.4 litre (216.4 fl.oz) 24-hour collection urine sample was that I was drinking way too much. At the levels I was drinking I had developed a false sense of thirst and I was at risk of becoming over hydrated and developing hyponatremia and hormone issues.

The Endocrinologist's advice? Cut back my water intake immediately and just "drink to thirst" instead. So now my recommendation is to drink when thirsty, but at least 2.4 litres (81 fl.oz) a day to ensure proper hydration. And that has to be pure clean water or herbal tea.

The reason is that even though tap or drinking water is monitored by the local Environmental Protection Agency (EPA) and certified as safe to drink, there are many existing minerals as well as some bacteria in them that can damage our health, skin and our appliances.

Most tap waters are chlorinated to prevent disease and many contain trace components of minerals, metals or bacteria at levels that are reportedly safe for consumption, including trace levels of aluminium as a result of the water treatment process.

Fluoride is added to most water supplies in an effort to control tooth decay, but many antipsychotic drugs contain fluoride and it is known as a neurotoxin - that is, toxic to nerve tissue.

There is evidence to support that fluoride only need to be used on the surface of teeth and then spat out, rather than ingested. There is also widespread concern that fluoride may interfere with thyroid function by interfering with the body's iodine receptors.

To hydrate yourself, pure or distilled water is a good option, but it doesn't contain any naturally occurring minerals, so you'll need to ensure that your dietary intake of vitamins and minerals is sufficient.

> *"You need to drink at least 2.4 litres of water each day just to maintain hydration status quo in the body, more if you're exercising."*

The best option is filtered water, but there are a vast array of filters on the market and many work better than others. There are three main processes of filtration: physical barrier, chemical process or biological process. Some filters use multiple processes to achieve their results.

Particulate Filters are the simplest and cheapest filtration method used to remove small amounts of suspended material from water. They can be used alone, or ahead of other water treatment devices and are also very effective at removing large bacteria and pathogens, like cysts such as Giardia and Cryptosporidium which are difficult to kill with low levels of chlorination.

Activated Carbon Filters are commonly found and relatively inexpensive. They work by absorbing organic contaminants that cause bad taste and odour and some also remove the by-products of chlorination; cleaning solvents and pesticides. The drawback is that these filters cannot remove metals such as lead and copper, nitrates, bacteria or dissolved minerals.

Ceramic Filters are porous allowing both water molecules, as well as smaller chemicals, to pass through. Ceramic filters block most microbes and if they have a colloidal silver lining it can help control bacterial build up. But these filters will not remove chlorine unless combined with an activated carbon filter.

Ion Exchange Units are good for hard water and remove calcium, magnesium and around 50% of fluoride. Whilst some models also remove radium and barium, they don't effectively remove any bacteria.

Reverse Osmosis (RO) Units are usually multi-stage filters that use activated carbon plus an ultra-fine reverse osmosis membrane and they excel at removing nitrates, sodium, fluorides, heavy metals, foul tastes, smells and colours. They can also reduce some pesticides, dioxins, chloroform and petrochemicals. The units are large and expensive, often require power to operate and produce up to 500% waste water. These are rarely seen in domestic situations and usually only used in commercial applications.

Distillation Units are generally used in commercial applications. They require electricity to boil water to vapour that is then collected and cooled. They produce the same end result as RO units except that pesticides and herbicides may be concentrated.

If you're concerned with the purity of your water, then invest in a good quality water filter. Melbourne's water supply is incredibly good with low levels of bacteria due to chlorination, but I still prefer the taste of filtered water and use a double under bench filtration system that employs particulate and activated carbon filters. And call me a water snob, but I take my own home filtered water everywhere!

However, if you enjoy tap water, stick with it. The health concerns are relatively minor compared with the increased benefits of drinking water instead of other beverages.

Whatever water or filtration you use it's really important that you consider the safety of container you store it in. Filtering the unwanted nasties out of it is great but if you then store it in a container that leaches other chemicals into it, what's the point?

If you're using plastic bottles (and they are convenient) then check the recycling symbol on your bottle. If it is a number 2 HDPE (high density polyethylene), a number 4 LDPE (low density polyethylene), or a number 5 PP (polypropylene), your bottle is fine to use and reuse.

Other numbers or un-numbered plastic bottles are probably not safe and can leach synthetic xenoestrogens into your water. These nasties are linked to breast cancer and uterine cancer in women, decreased testosterone levels in men, and are particularly devastating to babies and young children.

The best storage for your water is in ceramic or glass containers and out of direct sunlight.

Portion Sizes

Portion size is seriously out of control. With societal progress and the advent of restaurants, fast food outlets, and convenience food our portion control has literally gotten out of control.

I grew up with my parents telling me that I should finish all of the meat and vegetables on my plate at dinner, sometimes with the comment "there are children starving in Africa who'd love to have it" and failure to do so may result in no dessert. How many of you grew up in similar circumstances with parents and grand-parents from two post World War eras during which they experienced scarcity and food rationing to a degree that most of us will never know. It is easy to understand why they could not bear to see food wasted and there are many people today who still find it difficult, if not impossible to leave food behind or throw it away.

Fast food portion sizes and oversized meals in restaurants that all claim "big value for money" have taken their toll, stretched our stomachs and allowed us to forget the feeling of being sated without being stuffed.

A meal only needs to be between 200 and 400 calories, not the 500 to 1000 calories we often consume. It just needs to take the edge off hunger and provide energy for the next three to four hours. Anything more than that will automatically convert to sugar, be unexpended energy, which then converts into fat that deposits itself in all manner of unwanted areas in our bodies. We have lost all portion proportion and now our bodies are out of proportion. We need to re-educate our bodies and rediscover what a sensible portion size is.

> *"We have lost sense of portion proportion ~*
> *we need to re-educate our bodies*
> *about sensible portion sizes."*

A portion of protein does depend on your current weight, but when raw, should not be any bigger than your fist, roughly about 80g to 120g when cooked. The rest of your meal should be made up of vegetables, predominately leafy greens and low starch. One of the ways you can reduce your portion size at home without the need to weigh food is to buy a new place setting that has a smaller bowl or plate so less actually fits on it. And don't overload your plate – keep the food height fairly low.

The best way to re-educate yourself is have someone else prepare the food in a sensible meal size for you. This can be done by purchasing low fat ready-made meals from the supermarket, or subscribing to a home meal delivery plan. Whilst these are not ideal solutions for optimal nutritional value, they are incredibly beneficial short-term solutions to re-educate your body (and stomach) on appropriate quantities of food.

Tips for Eating Out

These days, with increased stress, increased work hours and reduced home time, we are eating out much more than ever before. The issue with eating out is that we can't tell what's actually in our food because we didn't prepare and cook it. Generally most restaurant food contains far more fat, sugar and salt than we would normally consume if we'd cooked at home and this is particularly the case with take away and home delivery, which has fast become the convenience food of our time.

Here are some ideas to help you make the best choices for you, so from an eating out perspective, you can have your cake and eat it too:

- Select restaurants where you know you can order healthy low fat options

- Avoid buffets and 'all-you-can-eat' specials

- Eat a little less at lunch (don't skip it though) if you're going out for a special dinner

- Eat a piece of fruit or have a glass of water with lemon 30 minutes before eating out

- Say "No" to the free bread or dinner roll

- Control portion size by ordering an entrée and a salad or side of steamed vegetables

- If you have to order a main then share it with a friend, or don't order anything else other than the main

- Always ask for the dressing on the side and carry your own dressing or a lemon just in case

- Avoid all fried food dishes and don't be afraid to ask how something's cooked if it's not clear.

- Ask if the main meat can be grilled, poached, baked or steamed rather than fried

- Never order chips, potatoes or rice. Ask for a salad instead.

- Don't go for bread-based dishes

- Request items be made without butter, flour or oil or added sauces

- If consuming alcohol set your limit before you start and stick to it.

- Ask for your soda or still water in a wine glass instead

- Don't order dessert, have a skinny latte or tea instead

- Carry sugar substitute to add to your coffee or tea

- Carry sugar free lollies just in case you need something sweet instead of dessert.

I practice all of these things regularly when I eat out. I also often carry a whole lemon in my handbag in case I'm confronted with a high calorie or creamy salad dressing. I'm also renowned for having my lime juice and soda in a wine glass and sometimes even adding some Stevia to it. It makes for a refreshing low calorie drink.

Gradually, over time, eating out will become easier and you'll become adept at making good healthy choices and avoiding bad ones.

> *"Over time, eating out will become easier and you'll become adept at making good healthy choices and avoiding bad ones."*

Creating New Habits

Habits are things you do automatically without really thinking through each step of the action simply because, in the past, you have done them so many times you've developed an inbuilt pattern for doing them. Things like putting your keys down when you come in the door, setting the alarm clock switch as you get into bed or flicking it off when it rings in the morning, driving a car (ever found yourself driving home the "wrong" way after moving house?), getting the mail and putting food in your mouth.

There are three main components to set a new habit. First you need to decide on the habit you want to create, and be specific with the requirements. You don't just say, "I want to drink more water". Instead you'd say, "I want to drink two litres of water every day".

Second, you need to set up a system of external reminders to prompt you to do it. Reminders can be messages, sticky notes, alarms, the help of friends, or simply by tying a string around your finger. Anything you can associate the desired new habit with. For example, I have three one litre water bottles that I fill every morning. I carry one around until it's finished then swap it over for another bottle. This triggers my mind to consciously and continually keep drinking.

Lastly, once you remember to perform the habit you actually need to perform the action, not just think it. It's great if I remembered to drink the water, but unless I actually drink the water then it doesn't mean anything and it doesn't start to create the new habit. Making the decision, being mindful about it and then getting into action many times is what will turn these behaviours into long term habits.

> *"Making decisions, being mindful about them*
> *and getting into repeated action*
> *turns behaviours into long term habits."*

Here are 16 techniques you can use to help you get there.

1. Start Simply

Don't try and recreate your world in one day. It's easier to focus on one change at a time. Make small incremental changes that build on each other. For example if you want to walk for an hour a day, start with 15 minutes and once that becomes regular (and easier) increase it to 30 minutes and so on until an hour a day becomes the "norm".

2. Write it Out

We've all heard of the stories of people who wrote their goals down, put them in the bottom drawer and forgot about them only to find months or years later that they'd come true. Writing your goals down makes them real. So, too, you should write down your habits to make the intangible real. Better still, don't stick them in a bottom drawer - instead stick them where you cannot fail to see them every day and keep them as a friendly reminder.

3. List the Cons

If you're up front with yourself and list the drawbacks to creating a new habit, then you can proactively deal with the issues so they become non-issues and non-reasons to quit.

4. List the Pros

Knowing the benefits of creating a habit can help counteract the cons and provide encouragement to continue. List all the possible benefits to your new habit – odds on they will far outweigh your cons.

5. Practice Daily

Doing the behaviour daily, rather than a couple of times a week, leads to greater repetition. That's one of the reasons that it's easier to make a daily action a habit than, say, going to the gym two or three times a week.

6. Don't Skip

Setting motivating reminders for yourself to perform your new habit is vital. Miss one day and then you'll miss the next, and soon you'll whittle away your chance to successfully create the habit.

7. Same Time, Same Place

Doing the habit at the same time and location each day can be a great association and reinforcement for it becoming a habit. I walk my dogs for at least an hour twice a day. We go to one of two parks at about the same time each morning, and again in the evening before bed – none of us feels right if we miss our daily walks!

8. Phone a Friend

Creating a new habit with a friend can make it fun and motivational. If you really don't want to go to the gym then having a gym buddy can help get you motivated to get there. When you set up your buddy system make an agreement with each other to support and "call" each other on any attempts to wangle out of it. Your buddy will get you motivated to get you back on track and, although you may hate their guts for making you do it. But afterwards you'll be glad they did.

9. Role Model Magic

Not unlike 'phoning a friend', getting a role model can be in important motivator. Studies have shown that the behaviour of the role model can 'wear off' onto you. So if you hang out with a smoker and you're trying to quit smoking it's probably not going to be an overly successful venture. So, too, if you're getting a gym buddy you should ensure that they are physically in the same or better shape that you, not worse.

10. Try a Trigger

Triggers, or prompters, can take all manner of forms and are fantastic reminders. A song, snapping your fingers, the list goes on. I sometimes use a rubber band around my wrist to remind me to stop doing the 'something' I don't want to do. A quick flick of it when the undesirable thought pops into my head snaps me back to my senses. Find a trigger that works for you.

11. Commit to a Month

A habit is much easier to sustain after you've been doing it for three or four weeks. Make a commitment to yourself that you'll play full tilt 100% for the next month to establish your desired habit.

12. Eliminate Temptation

If the habit you're trying to create is to stop doing something, like smoking, then make sure you clean your environment and remove any temptations that may be around. Making it harder for yourself to get to the undesirable item in the first place is paramount to supporting your new habit.

13. Substitute It

If your habit is to give something up, then you need to consider replacing it with something else that's supportive of your new habit. For example if you're giving up your usual relaxing time in front of the television to exercise, then you might want to include another relaxing activity like meditation. This will ensure that the subconscious is adequately looked after.

14. Instant Perfection

To expect instant perfection is to set yourself up for failure. It can take several attempts and a lot of persistence to develop that habit. If you fall off the habit horse, then dust yourself off and jump right back on.

15. Monitor Self Talk

Reminding yourself that you can do something is helping to set yourself up for success. Positive self-talk is a great way to motivate yourself and change your beliefs but it can be easier said than done. If you find you're telling yourself you can't do something then follow it with a "yet, but" statement – "I can't do it yet, but soon I will be able to".

> *"Follow 'I can't' statements with 'yet, but' statements to change your self-talk and perception."*

16. Set Rewards

Before you start a new habit identify four rewards you can give yourself (one a week) for completing the new habit each day for a full week. Make sure the rewards support, not undermine your desired new habit. At the end of each week, provided you have successfully undertaken your new habit each day then give yourself the reward. This will reinforce your positive behaviour, help set your new habit and each week will become easier.

Key Learnings

What are the main three reasons diets don't work?

1. _______________________________

____

2. _______________________________

____

3. _______________________________

____

What are the five most important things you've learned about nutrition (food, vitamins and supplements)?

1. _______________________________________

____

2. _______________________________________

____

3. _______________________________________

____

4. _______________________________________

____

5. _______________________________________

____

What five changes are you going to make to your food?

1. ____

____

2. ____

____

3. ____

____

4. ____

____

5. ____

____

What three changes are you going to make to the drinks you consume?

1. _______________________________________

____

2. _______________________________________

____

3. _______________________________________

____

What three things can you do to ensure you eat healthily when eating out?

1. _______________________________________

____

2. _______________________________________

____

3. _______________________________________

____

What three new habits are you going to create starting today?

1. ____

____

2. ____

____

3. ____

____

7. Get Your Body Right

Exercise? Yeah, right. I can hear all of your excuses right now. "I don't have any time or energy to do any exercise. I'm overweight to begin with, so what sort of exercise would possibly have any benefit for me. Perhaps I'll skip this chapter..."

Sounds like me when I weighed over 143kg (315 lbs) and whether it sounds like you now or not, keep reading.

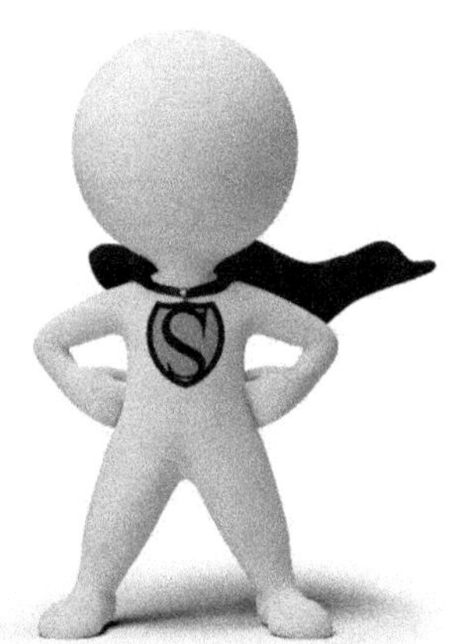

I know many of you don't really feel like doing any exercise, you're tired and may already be struggling with moving around and getting everything done in a day. I know how you're feeling – remember I was there. But please don't avoid this chapter! There is so much to be learned and even the smallest change can have an enormous impact on your health and weight loss.

In this chapter together we're going to look at why increasing activity is so important. We're going to check the pros and cons of cardio versus weight training and we're going to search far and wide for every possible option to increase your metabolism – in fact I'm going to share 16 techniques with you.

First you need to understand a few things.

Basal Metabolic Rate

Your Basal Metabolic Rate (BMR) is the amount of energy your body uses each day at rest. So basically it's just the amount all of your vital organs use - the heart, lungs, nervous system, kidneys, liver, intestine, sex organs, muscles, and skin. These functions generally comprise the majority of your calorie expenditure – even if you do a lot of exercise.

Your BMR increases from the time you are born until about two years of age, and then (unfortunately) declines every year thereafter except during puberty. So yes, as you get older, your metabolism drops, but then we all kind of knew that, didn't we?

It's good to understand what your current BMR is so that you understand the impact activity will have on it. There are a number of BMR formulae and each has its pros and cons. The main issue with all of the formulae is that they are based on body weight, and do not take into account the difference in metabolic activity between lean body mass and body fat. Lean body mass is far more metabolically active than body fat, which requires very few calories too be sustained.

> *"Body fat requires very few calories*
> *to be sustained unlike lean body mass*
> *which is far more metabolically active."*

The best formula to approximate your BMR (it's not an exact science) is a formula by Mifflin et al and can be shown as:

$$P = \left(\frac{10.0m}{1\ \text{kg}} + \frac{6.25h}{1\ \text{cm}} - \frac{5.0a}{1\ \text{year}} + s \right) \frac{\text{kcal}}{\text{day}}$$

where s = +5 for men, and -161 for women.

Using this formula, for example, a 55 year old woman weighing 130 lb (59 kg) and 5 feet 6 inches (168 cm) tall would have a BMR of 1204 kcal per day at rest, and between 1.2 and 1.9 times this amount depending on how active she was.

There are four main factors that affect your Basal Metabolic Rate. The first is body composition. Men naturally have a higher BMR than women because they have more lean body mass as well as more muscle mass, both of which are more metabolically active.

Women, unfortunately are disadvantaged on this one, not only because they generally have lower BMRs, but also because they generally have a higher level of body fat. Women's BMRs are at least 5% lower than men (and yes this is exactly the reason men can eat more calories than women). The good news is that women (and men) can increase their BMR by increasing their amount of muscle mass by practicing resistance training. More on this soon.

Following on from this, the second impact on BMR is your body condition, or level of fitness. An athlete would have a higher BMR than a non-athlete. As fat, lean body mass and fitness levels are all intertwined, it also goes that your fitness level has a lot to do with your BMR, particularly when at rest. Gradually getting fitter will gradually increase your BMR.

> *"Gradually getting fitter will gradually increase the amount of calories you consume at rest."*

The last major impactors on your BMR are the hormones the body secretes. The adrenal gland secretes epinephrine which gives you a short two to three hour BMR boost. The thyroid function is closely linked to BMR with hyperthyroidism giving you a 50% - 75% BMR increase and hypothyroidism resulting in a 30% decrease.

Other less important factors are sleeping too much and under nutrition - both will reduce your BMR up to 20%. BMR increasers are pregnancy (20%) and smoking (10%) although smoking is not recommended (but you can understand why so many people smoke to gain the benefits of an appetite suppressant as well as a BMR increase, despite playing Russian roulette with their lives).

The final two influencers of BMR are body temperature and environmental temperature. Every 0.55°C (1°F) increase in body temperature can result in up to a 7% increase in BMR. And environmentally the surrounding temperature can have an impact, extreme heat and cold both increasing BMR with BMR being at its lowest at about 26°C (78°F).

Increase Activity

Okay, so now you understand your BMR we can start discussing increasing your day to day activity.

Staying mobile and active well into your senior years will ensure that you stay more youthful, keep your body age down, maintain flexibility and reduce the risk of injury.

Not everyone can just jump feet first into a whole lot of exercise. If you've not partaken in exercise recently (or at all) then this section is for you. In increasing your activity all you need to do is to move more – whatever you can manage.

> *"The key is to just move more ~ do as much as you can easily and safely."*

Whether you're 16 or 60 going on 80, walking with a stick or wheelchair bound, there's a range of activities you can do that will help improve your situation. You may not see the results immediately, but gradually with small incremental changes you'll change the energy balance to build and maintain lean muscle while burning and losing fat at the same time. Eventually you'll notice your clothes are looser, your waistline is smaller and your energy levels are higher.

A lot of these activities depend on your physical size and current fitness level so I have categorised the exercise levels via your Body Mass Index.

BMI	% Body Fat	Exercise Type
> 45	> 45	Low Cardio Do not exercise to start with, focus solely on dietary control and moving more.
> 40 and < 45	> 35 and < 45	Medium Low-Impact Cardio Increase cardio by waking faster and longer, and aim to increase your target heart rate over time.
> 30 and < 40	> 30 and < 35	High Cardio Start interval jogging, or pursue other forms of exercise including swimming and push your heart rate higher.
> 25 and < 30	> 20 and < 30	Toning High Cardio plus Resistance Training
> 19 and < 25	> 15 and < 20	Maintenance Reduced number of sessions of cardio / resistance

Whatever your level, aim to move a little more in your day. Park further away from the shopping centre, and take the stairs instead of the lift. Walk to the shops or post office, instead of driving. Wear a pedometer or fitness tracker to track your step count, so you can gradually increase it.

If you are particularly big and find it hard to move, focus on low impact exercises such as swimming, aqua aerobics, walking and biking. If you are disabled, use a walking stick or are wheelchair bound, then consider doing upper body exercises – good old fashioned arm twirls and jumping jacks (without the jumping). There are a range of creative things you can do if only you put your thinking cap on. Gradually over time you'll be able to increase your movements and do more.

Go to **www.HalfTheWomanIWas.com** and click on the **VIP** tab for a *Customised Exercise Plan* that's just right for you.

Cardio vs Resistance

There is much controversy over which form of exercise is best. Cardiovascular exercise comprises regular aerobic exercise that forces your lungs to process more oxygen with less effort; your heart to pump more blood with fewer beats; and the blood supply directed to your muscles to increase, thereby increasing the endurance and efficiency of your body. Cardio exercise also increases weight loss (via energy expended); improves muscle health and mental functioning; increases stamina and your life span; as well as improving your immune system and reducing disease.

Resistance training may seem intimidating, but weight training can be done at a gym on large pieces of expensive equipment, or more simply, at home with free weights or resistance bands. Resistance training helps tone muscles, increase strength and muscular endurance, maintain lean body mass, decrease the risk of osteoporosis, develop coordination and balance, prevent injuries resulting from weak muscles and develop self-confidence.

The risks of cardio can include sprains, strains, stress fractures, arch and foot pain, heel spurs, Achilles tendon problems, calf pain and shin splints, particularly with high impact cardio. For this reason lower impact cardio exercises that get your heart rate up while being gentle on your joints are recommended. Stretching before and after exercise is a great way to improve flexibility and reduce the chance of injury. Dehydration prevents the body from functioning properly and can lead to poor brain function, kidney failures and coma, so it's important to drink plenty of water during the day as well as during and after exercise.

Resistance training can be much more difficult to perform accurately and safely. Without proper lower back support, or strong back and abdominal muscles there can be a risk of injury when performing certain free weight exercises such as squats, or standing overhead barbell presses. This can be minimised with adequate supervision and guidance.

Cardio is not better than resistance training, or vice versa - each will give good results. However, synergistically they work together to provide greater results than either individual one. So, for maximum results it's best if you combine the two and perform a mixture of cardio and resistance training.

> *"To achieve maximum results perform a mixture of cardio and resistance training each week."*

To get a copy of my *Resistance Training Program* simply head to **www. HalfTheWomanIWas.com** and click on the **VIP** tab.

Stretching is a Must

Stretching gently before and, particularly, after exercise has incredible beneficial effects. Stretching lengthens muscles and improves their tissue elasticity and flexibility. If done correctly, stretching will help prevent injuries and increase athletic performance.

Stretching tips:

- Start slowly with gradual exercises that mobilise all the joints to allow the body's natural lubrication (synovial fluid) to protect the surface of your bones at these joints.

- Warm up your body prior to stretching, so as to improve the blood flow around your body and make your muscles more supple.

- After exercise, slowly bring your heart rate down by first walking before you begin stretching, so as to prevent cramps and dizzy spells.

- Taking a hot bath or shower directly after exercise and before stretching can help relax the muscles

- Never bounce whilst you stretch. Instead hold the stretch for 30 to 50 seconds until you feel the muscle loosen off, then repeat for a further 15 seconds.

- Remember that during each stretch you should usually feel some slight discomfort, which is the muscle stretching, however you should stop immediately if you feel any severe pain.

- During each stretch don't hold your breath. Remember to breathe steadily and rhythmically.

For my *Stretching Guide* visit **www.HalfTheWomanIWas.com** and click on the **VIP** tab.

Maximise your Metabolism

Your metabolism is your furnace – it's what keeps your body going. Our metabolism (without exercise or movement) is responsible for burning up to 60% of the calories we consume each day.

The basic biology lesson is that the metabolism can be explained by a series of complex chemical reactions that must occur in every living organism in order for it to live. These reactions combine so that organisms can grow, maintain their structure, respond to their environment and reproduce.

> *"Your metabolism is your furnace ~*
> *learn how to feed it*
> *and it'll burn up your excess fat."*

Metabolism is broadly divided into two categories. Catabolism is destructive in that it breaks down organic matter into the energy components that can be used by anabolic reactions. Anabolism is constructive and uses energy to form the building blocks of cells such as proteins and nucleic acids.

Most organisms exist in constantly changing environments (stress, warmth, cold, etc.) and to maintain homeostasis, or the status quo for the body's internal biological stability, the body's metabolism automatically adjusts to accommodate any change in environment.

Those born and blessed with a high metabolism mean they naturally burn calories at a higher rate and are much less likely to put on weight regardless of what they eat. We all have a skinny girl nemesis: "How does she eat all that and stay so thin?" But the truth is there are also many people with such high metabolisms they are cursed because of the volume of food they must eat in order to keep weight on. I know, those of us cursed with a slow metabolism wish we had that problem!

A slow metabolism is usually made worse by eating too much food, eating the wrong combination of foods that don't support your digestive system, and a lack of physical activity. But even if you have a slow metabolism there's good news – it can be sped up using the following 16 techniques.

Technique 1: Increase Protein

Protein takes more energy to burn up, meaning it has a higher thermic effect than other nutrients like fats, sugars and starchy carbohydrates. In fact up to 25% of the calories of protein are consumed in its digestion and absorption. Protein is also essential for the growth and repair of the body's cells. Lastly, protein makes you feel full quicker and for longer than carbohydrates, which promote hunger. Just don't overdo it on the protein intake – more is not better and a diet that is too protein heavy will yield huge weight loss in the first few days but in the process it can place significant stress on your organs leading to health problems.

Technique 2: Increase Nutrients

Vitamins and minerals are essential to bodily function. Vitamin deficiency can lead to various medical issues (refer to the sections on Vitamin and Mineral RDIs). Overdosing on vitamins can also cause medical issues, so eating nutrient rich foods is all about balance. Bottom line – fresh is best, including fruits, vegetables, eggs, lean meats. Nuts and low fat dairy.

Technique 3: Focus on Fibre

Eating high fibre carbohydrates like fruits, vegetables and whole grain products makes you feel fuller for longer. Fibre rich foods are more difficult to digest than simple carbohydrates that rapidly convert to sugar, raising your blood sugar level and making you feel lethargic. Foods that are high in fibre are generally also lower in calories, and they also have a greater thermic effect. But as with all of these techniques, balance is key. Excessive fibre consumption can cause gastric issues including bloating, constipation and diarrhoea.

> *"Bottom line ~ fresh is best combined with foods that are high in fibre and have a greater thermic effect to help you burn fat quicker."*

Technique 4: Spice Up Your Life

Adding some spices to your cooking (chillies, curries, pepper, cayenne) can increase your metabolism by increasing your body temperature for a while after eating. Several metabolism specialists recommend a morning drink upon waking, made of the juice of a lemon with an equal quantity of warm water, half a teaspoon of cayenne and a teaspoon of honey. Again a little of these spices added to your dishes is the key – over consumption can lead to irritable bowel, heartburn and stomach ulcers.

Technique 5: Include Metabolism Boosting Foods

Metabolism boosting foods include green tea, black tea, capsicum or hot peppers, black pepper, ginger, mustard, coconut oil, asparagus, spinach, fish, poultry, eggs, fresh beans, broccoli, grapefruit, raw rolled oats and raw nuts. Each of these foods contains a metabolism booster so include as many of these foods as you can in your daily diet.

Technique 6: Eat Breakfast

Breakfast is literally that – a break from a fast of 12 hours or more. If you skip breakfast your metabolism can go into starvation mode, it will start to slow down and you'll begin to feel lethargic. Eating a good balanced breakfast within 30 minutes of waking can be critical in enrolling your metabolism to help achieve your goals.

Technique 7: Eat More Often

Research has showed that eating smaller meals more frequently can boost your metabolism. It takes about three hours for the energy in the food you eat to be exhausted, which is often why people start to either get hungry or tired after this period of time. The three square meals a day rule doesn't work for everyone. Breaking your three meals into four or five smaller meals spaced out at regular intervals can help maintain your energy levels and minimise bloating and digestive problems. But all your food should be consumed within a maximum 12 hour window, to facilitate a 12 hour fast overnight (e.g. 8pm until 8am daily).

Technique 8: Eat Earlier

Breakfast and lunch should be your main meals, with dinner being your lightest meal. Carbohydrates (even complex ones) should be avoided after lunch, and dinner should consist of lean meat and/or vegetables. It's best not to eat after 8pm or any later than three to four hours before bedtime. Giving your body this break from eating allows the food you've eaten to be burned while you're moving around rather than just heading for your hips as you sleep. This also means you'll be eager for breakfast when you wake up in the morning.

Technique 9: Don't Starve

Whilst it's generally accepted that in order to lose weight you need to reduce your calorie intake, dropping calories too fast or too low can have a disastrous effect by putting your metabolism into starvation mode. Ensure that you keep your daily calories above 1000, or higher, depending on how much you weigh and how much weight you have to lose.

Technique 10: Hydrate

Our bodies are made up of 70% water. Water is lost from our bodies at an average rate of 100mls per hour, and higher if exercising. As a result it's vital that we drink at least 2.4 litres of pure water every day. I highly recommend that you invest in a double filtration water filter that removes unwanted impurities. This will also help with the taste (pure water actually tastes almost sweet) but if you're still having trouble drinking plain water add some lemon to it. Visit **www.HalfTheWomanIWas. com** and click on the **VIP** tab access the *Resources Directory* for more information.

Technique 11: Avoid Alcohol

Yes, you knew this one was coming. Alcohol not only dehydrates the body but it's full of simple carbohydrates that quickly convert to high blood sugar. Further, excessive alcohol intake reduces the body's ability to absorb nutrients from those nutrient rich foods you're eating. Alcohol is not strictly taboo, but no more than two standard drinks on any one day and no more than four standard drinks each week if you want to get to your goal. And for every glass of alcohol you should consume some additional water to counteract its effect.

Technique 12: Cut out Caffeine

Like alcohol, caffeine also dehydrates the body. If you desperately need your coffee fix then consider alternate sources of caffeine such as guarana to wean yourself off this addictive substance. Part of the issue with having a coffee is it's not necessarily about having the coffee – it's about the socialisation. So if you fit into this category then try switching beverages to green or herbal tea instead. And again whilst caffeine is not strictly taboo, don't consume more than one standard shot of coffee on any one day and no more than five standard shots each week if you want to get to your goal. Switch out the full fat milk for low fat, and switch any sweetener for a low or no calorie version. And for every cup of coffee, you need to consume some extra water to counteract its effect.

Technique 13: Keep Moving

Moving around is one of the best ways to keep your metabolism up. It's the little extra activities that count like parking further away in the shopping centre car park. It's also important to monitor your progress daily so invest in a fitness tracker and aim for 10,000 steps each day.

Technique 14: Get Fit

Your metabolism is also affected by regular high intensity cardiovascular exercise (the kind that makes you sweat and pant). This activity not only burns calories while you do it, but physical activity also keeps your metabolism elevated for a few hours after the activity is finished. It's a double benefit, so work on getting your level of fitness up slowly by partaking in your favourite activity a few times a week.

Technique 15: Build Muscle

A kilogram of muscle burns three times as many calories at rest as a kilogram of fat. Resistance training will increase your lean muscle mass and therefore your metabolism. Partaking in a proper resistance training program three times a week and combining it with good nutrition will reduce fat and increase the amount of calories burnt whilst resting.

> *"Moving around more and performing resistance training are two of the most effective ways to speed up your metabolism."*

Technique 16: Helpful Supplements

Chances are that in your journey you will be expending more energy than you intake (that's the whole point!) and this can lead to tiredness or fatigue. Supplements that mimic substances the body naturally produces for energy production can be helpful in alleviating fatigue.

They include:

- Co-enzyme Q10, also known as CoQ10, which supplies energy to muscles

- L- Carnitine, which is responsible for the transport of fats from storage to energy conversion areas

- NADH (Nicotinamide Adenine Finucleotide), which helps cells convert food into energy

- Green Tea extract helps regulate blood sugar and aids digestion among other benefits.

It can also be helpful to get your thyroid tested. The thyroid controls how quickly the body uses energy, makes proteins, and it controls how sensitive the body should be to other hormones. Getting the thyroid balance right is very important.

An over active thyroid (hyperthyroidism) produces too many thyroid hormones and can lead to increased appetite, palpitations, excess sweating, diarrhoea, weight loss, muscle weakness and unusual sensitivity to heat. An under active thyroid (hypothyroidism) is the underproduction of thyroid hormones with typical symptoms of abnormal weight gain, tiredness, baldness and cold intolerance. Hypothyroidism is the most common thyroid problem for those who are overweight.

Even if your test returns in the 'normal' range your thyroid may still be under active and you may benefit from an iodine supplement. High potency iodine supplements are difficult to obtain locally. Low dose kelp concentrations are usually available locally, but you may have to get high potency supplements from overseas, which is relatively easy these days. Visit **www.HalfTheWomanIWas.com** and click on the **VIP** tab to access the *Resources Directory* for more details.

Survive Stress

In our modern day lives we are all plagued by stress, and for many people a small amount of stress is a useful motivator. However when we continue to experience a state of ongoing physiological arousal (and please get your mind out of the gutter right now) stress becomes chronic and harmful.

We are plagued by an abundance of stress that presents itself in many different forms and comes from many different sources: work, family, financial, health, social and self-imposed. The reality is that for most of us stress in our modern lives has become chronically present - it is not only one of the main reasons for weight gain but it is a silent and very tragic killer. It can also cause mental and emotional symptoms including anxiety, depression, allergies, dizziness, headache, heart palpitations, environmental sensitivity, impaired coordination and impaired immunity.

In Neolithic times stress was a useful attribute for protection and life preservation - the fight or flight reaction driven by the powerful hormones adrenalin and cortisol (think "tiger going to eat man, man better run fast"). This hormone reaction changes the way our bodies function, for we start to behave as though we're in danger. Too much stress all at once or continual, ever-present lower level stress in our lives can create excess hormone presence and can eventually lead to insulin resistance and weight gain.

When the body is experiencing stress it excretes a corticotrophin-releasing hormone and adrenalin, that in turn stimulate the release of cortisol from the adrenal cortex. Cortisol, a glucocorticoid, then stimulates the release of glucose into the bloodstream, which can, in periods of chronic stress, produce an excessive release of insulin (a fat-storage hormone). Cortisol increases appetite, particularly for fatty, salty and sugary carbohydrates. It slows the metabolism, while the excessive release of insulin raises blood sugar, leading to mood swings and fatigue. Insulin also gives the body the message to store fat in the abdomen, overriding the message from the adrenalin to burn the fat instead. And hey presto, you gain weight. Simply put, excessive stress helps you put on extra weight and keep it on; so it is important to find ways to minimise the amount of stress you experience.

> *"Excessive stress can cause weight gain ~*
> *find ways to minimise your stress levels."*

Eating carbohydrates, particularly simple ones, also stimulates production of serotonin, the brain's mood-calming neurotransmitter, and one gets a feeling of happiness and relaxation. But this feeling is only short lived, until the carbohydrate rush is over, and the cycle begins again. Eating complex carbohydrates not only ensures that the brain gets enough fuel, but the resulting slow release of sugars into the blood stream ensures that both insulin and serotonin are released gradually instead of an unhealthy rush.

Long term, this stress response affects insulin regulation and alters glucose metabolism and fat storage and it's not for the better, as it can lead to type 2 diabetes and other medical issues. But stress should not be considered in isolation - the incorrect function of other organs, such as the hypothalamus, pituitary, thyroid, adrenal and sex glands can also have an impact lowering your basal metabolic rate and causing obesity.

Okay so we get it – stress is bad. But how do we lower it?

How do we get our bodies working for us and not against us?

It's not so easy if you have a stressful job, a mortgage to pay and a family to look after. You can't just run away or quit. But there are some things you can do to help lower your stress levels, reduce your cortisol levels, manage and treat short-term stress and stress-related illnesses and prevent some of the precursors to weight gain.

If you want to find out how stressed you are then head to **www. HalfTheWomanIWas.com** and click on the **VIP** tab and take the *Stress Test* and get your free report.

LIFESTYLE CHANGES

If your job is stressful then you need to employ **stress management techniques**. Schedule your day, be proactive rather than reactive. Bulk reply to your emails several times a day and set aside chunks of time to complete more important time consuming tasks without interruption. You'll be far more productive.

Take breaks. I was very bad at this, often sitting at my computer for hours on end only getting up when my bladder was literally about to burst! Take a break every hour even if it's just for a few minutes to catch your breath or get a cuppa. When you return more refreshed after your break you will be much more productive, which will more than make up for the five minutes you've taken off.

Practice the **Pareto principle**, and if something's really important someone will remind you. I used to think everything was critically important and only I could fix things. I was taking on far too much and putting myself under self-imposed pressure and responsibility. It's taken me a long time to realise that I need to have strict boundaries. If it's not my role I don't take it on – I push back or delegate. Yes, if you're like me, you will notice that things won't get done as quickly or as accurately; but does it really matter as long the job does get done and you have less stress as a result?

Do you practice **emotional eating**? Increased stress levels increase cortisol levels and make you crave unhealthy food and eat more than you normally would. When you go to snack or eat, make sure you really are hungry. Before eating drink a full glass of water, or a cup of herbal tea and then wait 10 or 20 minutes. Nine out of 10 times the urge to eat will subside as you are not actually hungry.

Too busy to cook? Fast food is full of unhealthy fats, sugar, salt and toxins that your body has to work harder to get rid of. Don't stress your body out by filling it with these nasties – you'll be paying a far higher price than the cost of the food. Making a quick healthy salad doesn't take much time when you know how. If you really don't have time then grab pieces of apple, carrot and celery and snack on them.

Exercise is one of the most beneficial activities to lower unwanted stress levels, even though it may cause a small amount of stress on your body performing it. While exercise may be the last thing on your mind, even taking just a 10 minute walk will greatly reduce the effects of stress. High impact or high intensity exercise involve good stressors on the body and will result in even more stress reduction benefits afterwards. So get outside in the sunshine, feel the grass underneath your feet or partake in the horizontal mambo. Don't think about it - just do it!

"Minimise the unwanted stress in your life but don't stress out about reducing stress — it's counterproductive!"

SUPPLEMENTS

Studies have shown that a combination of the 11 B-group vitamins (particularly B, B_3, B_6 and B_{12}) aids the support of a healthy central nervous system and brain. If B vitamins are deficient in the food, using a B-complex supplement may assist.

Vitamin C, an important anti-stress antioxidant, can reduce corticotrophin-releasing stress hormone levels in the bloodstream, thereby allowing the immune system to work more effectively to combat stress.

Herbal Products

Some of the following products may be useful. Remember to refer to the manufacturer's instructions for doses, limits and side effects.

Relora is a plant-based extraction from the Magnoliaceae plant family particularly effective at reducing anxiety, irritability and nervousness without being sedating and with potential antidepressant properties.

The **Kava** plant contains kavalactones that seem to act on the limbic system, promoting relaxation, sleep and rest by changing the way the limbic system modulates emotional processes. Kava preparations are approved medicines in several European countries for treating nervousness, anxiety, minor depression and restlessness, whilst improving vigilance, sociability, memory and reaction time.

Ginseng comes in several different forms that have been used to promote a variety of health benefits in India and Asia for hundreds of years.

Panax Ginseng (Panax quinquifolium) is said to act in the hypothalamus and pituitary glands to increase the body's stress coping ability, including physiologic, emotional and endogenic (external) toxin stress, thus lowering the body's vulnerability to illness.

Ashwagandha (Withania somnifera) root, also known as winter cherry or Indian ginseng augments mental and physical functioning, improving the ability to learn, decreasing stress and fatigue and is used to treat insomnia, nervousness and restlessness.

St John's Wort is a persistent gentle nerve tonic, well known anti-depressant and a good choice for moderate depression and menopause. It's been prescribed in Germany for many years but can interfere with prescription medicines such as anti-depressants, hypertensive (high blood pressure) drugs, warfarin, AIDS medication and the contraceptive pill.

Rhodiola (Rhodiola rosea), or Arctic root, is a traditional medicine from China, Serbia and the Ukraine said to improve the nervous system, combat depression, enhance immunity, increase exercise capacity, improve memory and heighten energy levels.

Holy Basil (Ocimum sanctum), also known as tulsi or sweet basil, has been long used in Eastern and Middle Eastern countries to counteract stress by balancing blood corticosteroid levels.

FOODS

Almonds	High in unsaturated fat but a good source of Vitamin B2 and E, magnesium and zinc, which fights the free radicals associated with stress
Avocados	High in monounsaturated fats and potassium to lower blood pressure
Beef	Best meat for high levels of zinc, iron, and B vitamins to help level your mood
Blueberries	Rich in antioxidants and Vitamin C
Broad Beans	Rich in L-dopa which raises your mood, may help control high blood pressure and is used in the treatment of Parkinson's disease
Dried Apricots	Rich in magnesium and a natural muscle relaxant
Green Vegetables	High in the necessary vitamins to replenish our bodies in times of stress
Low Fat Dairy	High in antioxidants and vitamins B2 and

	B12, as well as protein and calcium
Oranges	Rich in vitamin C, boosts the immune system, reduces stress and returns blood pressure and cortisol to normal levels
Pistachios & Walnuts	Help to lower blood pressure
Salmon	High in omega-3 fatty acids, protect against heart disease and prevents cortisol and adrenaline from peaking
Soy & Soy Products	High in protein, B vitamins, calcium and magnesium but also affect your hormones so best avoided all together.
Spinach	High in magnesium reducing the possibility of migraine headaches and fatigue
Sweet Potatoes	High in beta-carotene, other vitamins and fibre and can satisfy the stress-induced urge for carbohydrates
Tuna	High in vitamins B6 and B12, low fat and high protein
Turkey	Contains L-tryptophan, an amino acid that triggers the release of serotonin and produces a calming effect

Whole Grains	Bulger wheat, quinoa, oats and brown rice are rich in B vitamins, fibre and supply serotonin producing carbohydrates that don't cause blood sugar levels to spike

Nurture Your Body

This journey may initially be tough on your body. With a sudden change in routine comes a newfound connection with your body and things that you may have been previously unaware of may be brought to the forefront.

Fortunately there are over 80 types of natural therapies available. There is no one best therapy for the body. Each one offers the recipient an individual experience. It's a matter of trying the therapies that appeal to you and seeing which ones work.

Following is a list of therapies you may be interested in trying:

Acupressure	Chiropractic	Feng Shui
Acupuncture	Colonic Irrigation	Flower Essences
Alexander Technique	Colour Therapy	Hellerwork
Allergy Testing / Treatments	Core Energetics	Herbal Medicine
Animal Therapy	Counselling	Holistic Doctor
Antenatal Classes	Craniosacral Therapy	Homeopathy
Aromatherapy	Crystal Therapy	Hypnobirthing
Art Therapy	Cupping	Hypnotherapy
Ayurveda	Day Spas	Iridology
Beauty Therapy (Holistic)	Dietitian	Kinesiology
Biofeedback	Dorn Therapy	Laser Therapy
Biomesotherapy	Doulas	Life Coaching
Body Harmony®	Ear Candling	Live Blood Analysis
Bowen Therapy	EFT (Emotional Freedom Techniques)	Lymphatic Drainage
Brain Gym®	Energy Healing	Magnetic Field Therapy
Breathwork	Exercise Physiology	Massage
Buteyko Breathing Technique	Feldenkrais Method	Meditation

Men's Health	Podiatry	Spiritual Healing
Myofascial Release Therapy	Polarity Therapy	Sports Injury Therapy
Myopractic	Pranic Healing	Tai Chi
Myotherapy	Psychotherapy	Theta Healing
Natural Fertility Management	Qi Gong	Thought Field Therapy
Naturopathy	Reconnective Healing	Time Line Therapy®
Neuro Linguistic Programming	Reflexology	Touch for Health
Nutrition	Reiki	Traditional Chinese Medicine (TCM)
Osteopathy	Remedial Therapies	Trigger Point Therapy
Personal Training	Rolfing® or SI	Weight Loss
Physiotherapy	Shiatsu	Women's Health
Pilates	Sound Therapy	Yoga

Circle the Therapies you would like to explore further

I have tried many of these therapies including acupressure, acupuncture, allergy testing, aromatherapy, biofeedback, Bowen therapy*, breathwork, chiropractic*, counselling, cupping, day spas, EFT*, flower essences, herbal medicine, hypnotherapy, iridology, life coaching, lymphatic drainage, massage*, meditation*, myotherapy*, naturopathy, NLP*, nutrition, physiotherapy, Pilates*, podiatry, Qi Gong, reflexology, reiki, remedial therapies*, shiatsu, sports injury therapy, time line therapy, TCM* and yoga*. Those I continue to use regularly are asterisked.

In trying natural therapies it is important to find a reputable and qualified therapist. Refer to your natural therapies association and also ask whether the therapists have practice insurance.

Visit **www.HalfTheWomanIWas.com** and click on the **VIP** tab to access the *Resources Directory* for more details.

Key Learnings

What are the top three things you learned about your Basal Metabolic
Rate?

1. ____

____

2. ____

____

3. ____

____

What three things can you do, other than exercise, to be more active?

1. ____

   ____

2. ____

   ____

3. ____

   ____

What are the top three things you learned about cardio and resistance training?

1. _______________________________

____

2. _______________________________

____

3. _______________________________

____

How are you going to put these into practice?

____

____

____

____

What are the top three techniques you are going to use to increase your metabolism?

1. _______________________________________

____

2. _______________________________________

____

3. _______________________________________

____

What are the top three things you learned about stress and its impact on your weight?

1. ____

____

2. ____

____

3. ____

____

What five things are you going to do to reduce your stress levels?

1. _______________________________________

____

2. _______________________________________

____

3. _______________________________________

____

4. _______________________________________

____

5. _______________________________________

____

What three techniques or natural therapies are you going to use to nurture your body?

1. ____

____

2. ____

____

3. ____

____

8. Get Your Spirit Right

Oprah Winfrey said, "If you want to accomplish the goals of your life, you have to begin with the spirit". She also said "It isn't until you come to a spiritual understanding of who you are - not necessarily a religious feeling, but deep down, the spirit within - that you can begin to take control".

Don't skip this chapter because you think it's about religion – it isn't. Getting your spirit right is about getting your subconscious working for you, instead of against you. It's about being true to yourself, and clearing all of that unwanted baggage that's holding you back from being the real you!

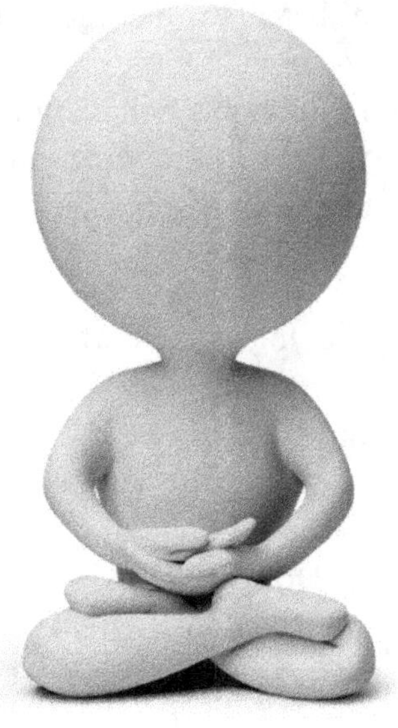

Whilst diet and exercise are two very important keys to this journey, getting your spirit aligned to your body and mind is the third apex of this plan and it's crucial to getting long lasting results. It's also the area that most weight loss programs fail to address adequately, and one of the main reasons that people fail to reach their health goals.

> *"Getting your spirit aligned to your body and mind is the third apex crucial to getting long lasting results."*

So if it's not religion, what is the sprit? Basically the human spirit is comprised of human philosophy, psychology as well as religion – lots of big words and even bigger subject matter about life, the universe and everything, right? Oh yeah, and the answer is 42. But these three ideas of rational thought, behavioural understanding and ethical spirituality come together to form your spirit – or your belief system – and it is this that underpins your subconscious and creates your reality.

Imagine having a support system that automatically and effortlessly creates everything you ever wanted or dreamed of, one day at a time, without any struggle at all. Imagine for a minute how incredible that would be – that you would never have to worry again, you would just know that you are on your true purpose, on track and reaching your goals every day. Don't you want that? Don't you want life to be easy not a painful and frustrating daily struggle that seems to have no end? Instead, just easy breezy lemon squeezy. Can you believe, just for a minute, that it really is possible? Can you fathom that thought?

I'll let you into a secret - you can have it, you really can. But first you need to understand your spirit and how to communicate with it so that the two of you can work together – because right now your ship has no Captain and there's mutiny afoot. Your vessel will surely end up floating aimlessly at sea, run aground, or be shipwrecked on the reef if your life continues the way it has so far.

Remember you are on your own journey - sailing around the world single-handed which means you truly only have yourself to rely upon. You are both Captain and crew and if the journey fails it is you and only you who can be held responsible for the failure.

In Captaining a vessel, equipment like the sails, engine, navigation charts, radar and so on, is used to ensure a safe and successful journey – a Captain knows this. But a good Captain has great knowledge and skills and executes them to perfection. And a great Captain also understands his environment; can read the wind and the waves, the sun and the stars and instinctively navigates to the desired destination with the safety of his crew in mind and his vessel and equipment intact.

To get your spirit right, you'll need to get your Captain's license. If you've covered the first two sections you have the knowledge and the skills and you're two-thirds there. Now you need to learn how to read the environment, to listen to the whisper of the wind, understand the waves and their tides, read the sunrise, or sunset and navigate by the stars. Oh, and don't forget you'll need to get your vessel ship shape and clear any barnacles before you set off. So read on and let me help you become the best possible Captain you can be!

Are you Captain Material?

There are 10 main qualities to being a good Captain. Let's find out where you are currently compared with where you'd like to be by ranking, on a scale of 1 to 10 (with 1 being poor, or no skill at all and 10 being where you'd ideally like to be, el supremo, numero uno - with absolutely no room for improvement). Add up your scores and let's find out what sort of Captain you are right now.

1. Honesty

A Captain must be honest. Failure to be honest means your crew won't trust you. On this journey you are rowing your own boat, you are your own crew; so are you going to lie to yourself? A lack of trust leads to a lack of loyalty and mutiny. If you lie to yourself, your mind, body and spirit will mutiny, undermine your weight loss efforts and make you fail. Arthur C. Clarke says *"The best measure of a man's honesty isn't his income tax return. It's the zero adjust on his bathroom scale."* How honest are you with others? More importantly how honest are you with yourself? Can you look yourself in the mirror, gaze into your eyes and tell yourself exactly what you see? Can you be truthful about acknowledging where you are now and how you got there? Can you be really honest about the amount of work that's needed to get to your destination?

Your score out of 10

2. Responsibility

Making a good decision and taking the kudos for the positive outcome is easy. But can you take equal responsibility for the bad decisions that you've made? Good Captains don't pass the buck or blame others – they make decisions and deal with situations that arise, they take responsibility for the results. As a Captain, even if you delegate to someone else and they stuff it up, guess what? It's your fault! You overestimated their capability and you have to take responsibility for that and for the outcome. Are you willing and able to accept full responsibility for all of the decisions, good or bad, and the outcomes in your life? If you haven't in the past, are you willing to do this now?

Your score out of 10

3. Confidence

Captains must believe in their ability – they must be supremely confident, speak the truth and believe every word that they say. The crew can detect untruths at three paces and know when the wool is being pulled over their eyes. Dr Norman Vincent Peale, author of *The Power of Positive Thinking* says, *"Believe in yourself! Have faith in your abilities! Without a humble, but reasonable confidence in your own powers you cannot be successful or happy"*. So how confident are you? Is what you are saying congruent with your actions? Are you walking your talk? More importantly do you believe your talk in the first place? Or are you living a lie and fooling yourself that nobody else has a grasp of the real truth about you? How confident are you about achieving your health and wellbeing goals?

Your score out of 10

4. Enthusiasm

Enthusiasm and passion are infectious and incredible motivators. If a Captain is excited about the journey to a new foreign land, odds on that at least some of it will rub off on the crew and they'll be more willing to roll up their sleeves and help get there. Steve Maraboli, author of *Life, the Truth, and Being Free* says, *"Live your truth. Express your love. Share your enthusiasm. Take action towards your dreams. Walk your talk. Dance and sing to your music. Embrace your blessings. Make today worth remembering"*. How enthusiastic are you about your life? Are you just going through the motions, or are you breathless with excitement as you grab your life with both hands and yell "hang on for the ride"? Do you follow your passions, or are you struggling to find them? How enthusiastic are you about increasing your vitality?

Your score out of 10

5. Reliability

Imagine a ship with a Captain that never turns up to work, or doesn't do the things he says he will? Nobody likes an unreliable person, even if they're not a leader, and it leads to mistrust. *"The shifts of Fortune test the reliability of friends"* was once uttered by Roman philosopher Marcus Tullius Cicero. Are you a reliable person? Or are you just a fair-weather friend who blows in when you feel like it, or when you need something? How many times have said you're going to do something, and not done it? On this journey the person you most need to rely upon is yourself. Can you? Is your reliability out of integrity? Can you step up now and be reliable in your commitment to your health?

Your score out of 10

6. Patience

Don't underestimate the importance of patience. It's something I often get short of, particularly in the work place (not one of my best qualities!) But what I do try to remember is that people only go to work to do a good job and if they've made a mistake, then nine times out of 10 it's because my instructions weren't clear enough. As a Captain it's critical that you take the time to give clear and concise instructions that are not prone to misinterpretation. When mistakes occur you need to have the patience to work through them so your crew understands what you are trying to achieve. As you are your own crew, this means you need to have the courage and the patience to confront yourself with the mistake you have made and work through it to figure out the way to a good outcome. Aristotle was quoted as saying. *"Patience is bitter, but its fruit is sweet"*. How patient are you? With others? With yourself? How patient do you think you can be with yourself on your road to health and vitality?

> Your score out of 10

7. Decisiveness

When peril lays in the path ahead Captains can't sit on the fence – they need to make a fast decision based on the information they have at hand. The decision doesn't always need to be the right one, sometimes getting into action is better than no action at all – for you can always change direction on the move. Napoleon Hill, author of *Think and Grow Rich* says, *"The way to develop decisiveness is to start right where you are, with the very next question you face"*. Do you make decisions quickly and decisively, or do you labour over them while you slosh around in a sea of indecision and inaction? Do you contingency plan and ensure you are one step ahead of any disaster that may occur, ready to make the necessary decision at a moment's notice, or do you wait until the proverbial hits the fan? How willing are you to make the tough decisions about your weight loss?

Your score out of 10

8. Determination

Captains need to be determined to finish what they started, see it through to the end and keep their crew motivated to continue to completion. The determination, desire and will to succeed is paramount to success. American football coach Vince Lombardi says, *"The difference between a successful person and others is not a lack of strength, not a lack of knowledge, but rather a lack in will"*. This is echoed by major league baseball player Tommy Lasorda: *"The difference between the possible and the impossible lies in a person's determination"*. If you begin with the determination to succeed then the job is already half complete. When you set goals do you achieve them, or does your will to achieve wane in the face of obstacles? How determined are you to achieve your goals this time, and reach your destination?

Your score out of 10

9. Loyalty

Captains expect the utmost loyalty from their crew. But it's not a one way deal. In return, the crew expects loyalty from their Captain. At the heart of JRR Tolkien's *Lord Of The Rings* trilogy is a story of loyalty between Frodo and Sam. *"You can trust us to stick with you through thick and thin, to the bitter end. And you can trust us to keep any secret of yours, closer than you keep it yourself. But you cannot trust us to let you face trouble alone and go off without a word. We are your friends, Frodo"*. How loyal are you to others in your life? How loyal have you been to yourself? Are you willing to be your own best friend, through good times and bad, and see your journey through to the end?

Your score out of 10

10. Courage

The core concept of the entire Harry Potter series, courage, is by far the most important quality in a Captain. Captains can't be afraid of failure, and they need courage to stick to their convictions, or admit when they were wrong. Dr May Angelou wrote, *"Courage: the most important of all the virtues because without courage, you can't practice any other virtue consistently"*. How courageous are you? Are you courageous Captain material ready to steer your vessel into unchartered waters, to listen to the whisper of the wind, to understand the waves and the tides, to read the sunrise and sunsets and navigate by the stars? Are you ready for the challenge that lies ahead?

Your score out of 10

Now add up your score and let's see how you did.

Your total score out of 100

Look up your score in the following table to see how you did.

Your score

0-30

If you've really scored this low then we have a lot of work to do to get you to a Captain's status. Let's start by working on your confidence and courage and the rest will follow. Don't give up, read on and let's get you there.

31-50

Well you're not quite captain status, more like a senior deckhand, but at least you've got your sea legs and are ready to sail. Full marks though for honesty and integrity. In fact rescore yourself with 10 points for item 1 and jump to the next level. You deserve it.

51-75

Well done, you've attained First Mate status. The first mate makes the decisions whilst the captain is busy, and so is critical on this journey you're about to take. All the First Mate needs to do to become Captain is learn from him, keep reading and hone your skills. And if you were thinking you could kill the Captain and take his role even for just a minute then rescore yourself with 0 for items 5 and 9 and move down a grade.

76-90

Congratulations, you've reached the status of Captain. There's still room for improvement (there's always room for improvement) but you have the core traits necessary to lead your crew and your vessel on this journey. Good luck and safe passage!

90-100

If you scored this high then either you don't have a weight or health problem to resolve, or if you do, you need to now rescore yourself and lower your score to 0 for items 1 and 2 and move down at least one level.

The reality is all of these 10 characteristics are intertwined. Not one of them can exist without the other and any failure in one surely has an impact on many, if not all, of the others. Having done this exercise you now have an awareness of the areas you need to focus on and improve.

In my journey was I a good Captain? Did I stay on track, eating and exercising perfectly, all the time? Absolutely not. I probably started as First Mate. Some days I let my ship run aground, my train derail and my star-ship get stranded in the delta quadrant (occasionally on the verge of being assimilated by the Borg). But as I learned to be Captain I became more competent at preventing large errors of judgement and corrected small ones quickly in order to get back on course.

One more thing. Don't waste time or energy regretting, or lingering over any relapses – learn from them. Then put your Captain's hat back on and get on with the journey. Over time you will find it easier to stay on course.

Now that you have an understanding of the qualities to be a Captain, let's start honing your skills.

Nature's Whisper - Understanding Your Environment

A Captain needs to intrinsically understand and be in tune with his environment. Smelling the wind, listening to it and feeling it upon his face and body will enable a Captain to know which way to head and which course to plot. This intimate knowledge can also help a Captain avoid disaster by being able to determine if the wind is just a stiff breeze, or whether a storm is coming and a new course needs to be set to avoid disaster. Being in tune with all aspects of your environment, both the one inside you as well as external to you, is a skill you need to develop. But sometimes things are not as they seem and it can take extensive experience, or help from others, to determine fact from fiction.

On this journey you now need to reflect for a minute and give yourself a reality check. Is how you think the world works around you really how it works, or is it just your perception and something else is really happening? It's the experiences we have as we grow up that colour our perception of reality, that create the paradigm in which we live and through which we interpret the whole of our existence.

> *"Give yourself a reality check ~*
> *is what's going on your perception or reality?"*

Without getting too new age on you, as a child you are born with a unique understanding of the world around you – that everything and everyone is perfect, and love is the only thing that matters. But as you grow from a child and develop into an adult you have experiences along the way that change this original belief.

Think about it for a minute. Growing up, how many times did you have a negative experience change the way you perceive the world? Were you called names, told you weren't smart enough at school, or told you were bad or naughty for doing something that your parents didn't want you to do? All of these experiences, whilst they may seem benign, leave their mark on you and change the way you behave and not necessarily for the better.

There's a lot of research out there to support the general principle that what you think about yourself manifests into reality. This is based on the interpretive powers of the brain, trying to make sense of all the billions of stimuli and pieces of information it receives each day, most of which are filtered out automatically by a preconceived set of self-imposed criteria (otherwise you'd drop dead from overload).

For example, did you ever think that a particular car would be nice to own because it's unusual and there are so few of them on the road, only to be shocked days later when you start noticing how many of them are actually on the road? What! Did the car dealership just sell their monthly targets over the past three days? No, they didn't. You are seeing the cars because you programmed your brain to notice that car, so now you do. Simple, right?

So, too, your brain filters information to fit your own set of established beliefs, in fact it specifically seeks information to support your beliefs; in this way it becomes a self-fulfilling prophecy. "Thin people are superficial and mean" – if that's what you believe then time and time again you'll come across these sorts of people, have your belief reinforced and so continue to believe it. It can also prevent your subconscious from wanting to be thin by rationalising to itself that as thin people are mean, I'll stay fat because I don't want to be mean. And this all happens without you even knowing it as the result of experiences you have had in your past.

> *"Your brain filters and seeks information to support your beliefs and create a self-fulfilling prophecy."*

Don't try to fix this for now – just understand that your brain always tries to fit the pieces of the jigsaw together to make a picture and as it does it draws conclusions and tries to make sense, a whole picture of all of these individual experiences. Sometimes the conclusions your subconscious draws are not the ones you would come to at a conscious level. And therein lies the problem.

You are not the driver of your vehicle known as the body. Your subconscious is and you can't consciously change the direction it's going in. Some of the connections our subconscious makes are helpful and some instructions, or directives, it gives us aren't. In getting your spirit right it's important to investigate your own subconscious and determine if there is programming in there that is not supportive of your goals.

There's an interesting story of a woman that used to get a headache every time she drove through a pine forest. It turns out that as a child she was in a car accident that occurred in a pine forest and hit her head badly. She did not consciously realise that every time she drove through the pine forest her subconscious was manifesting a headache because it thought it had to – that was its reality; it had connected pine forests with having a headache.

So now think about all those failed diet attempts – realise that they don't mean than you can't succeed and reach your health goals. You can. You just need to do some fine tuning of your subconscious to get it supporting your goals.

How many connections has your subconscious brain made that prevent you losing weight? What are the beliefs you may have that are preventing you from being thin? Take a few minutes to write your thoughts down now.

Tides of Change - Believe and Achieve

Just as the gravity of the moon impacts the tides, the winds have a huge impact on the size of the waves. By reprogramming your subconscious you can learn to control the winds, reduce the waves and go with the flow of the moon's gravity to create smooth still waters that will speed up your journey. It might sound a bit 'out there', but it is true.

The power to create your dreams and to attain your goals comes from the choices you make and the actions you take, both of which are guided by your subconscious. Don't fool yourself that you can avoid making a decision, for the illusion of seeming to make no decision is still making a decision – it's just not doing you much good and certainly not helping you achieve your goal. So you can make the choice not to participate, not to set forward on your journey towards the destination you long to reach, or you can make a different choice and change your life.

I really do believe that for the most part we create or choose everything that happens to us. Even if it's something bad, it has happened to us as a result of our decision or indecision, often for a grander purpose. So we actually create our own reality. Neuro-Linguistic Programming (NLP) specialist Christopher Howard sums this up perfectly by saying, *"If there's a poisonous snake at my foot, or I just believe that there is, I will react the same way"*.

> *"We really do create our own reality by our thought, our beliefs and by our actions or inactions."*

So you may want to ask yourself whether you are on the action or reaction side of your reality. Do you act to make things happen, or just let things happen to you and then react? Are you the victim in your life, or the victor? Have you taken responsibility for where you are today, the decisions that led to your size, your shape, your health, your fitness and your wellbeing? Or do you have some reason or excuse for where you're at? Worse still, do you blame others?

If you are blaming others for your reality are you hiding behind being a victim of abuse and making that the reason for creating a wall of protective fat around yourself? All this decision has done is disempower you, give you an excuse to blame someone else for your weight predicament and undermine your goal to lose weight.

Ditch the belief. It's time to step up and accept that the reason you are the way you are is because you choose to be this way. The power to change your reality and take charge of your destination comes from taking full responsibility for your current state, and deliberately and consciously making decisions that lead you toward your destination. If you can't accept this position, then things are not going to change for you.

> *"The power to change your reality and take charge of your destination comes from taking full responsibility for your current state."*

All learning, behaviour and change occur in a way that is unconscious. When you truly learn something it transfers to the unconscious mind and becomes part of your whole. For example, when you first got into a manual car and you saw three pedals did you wonder whether this vehicle was built for an alien, or whether you were born missing a leg? Sure it was difficult and challenging at first but now that you have learned how to drive, when you get into a car to drive, do you think about the purpose and complicated timing of using those three pedals, or do you just drive because it has become automatic or a habit?

Automatic, subconscious behaviour cannot be consciously changed. If I were to say don't think of a pink poodle, what are you thinking of? You could think of something else now, but odds on that it was a two-step process and you thought of the pink poodle first and then consciously had to think of something else.

It's the same situation with conscious self-talk. If you are saying to yourself, "I can't lose weight," then guess what, you won't be able to.

The only way to change your results is to attack the issue on two fronts. First, change your conscious self-talk to positive supportive talk, and secondly to reprogram your subconscious and align it with your goals and desires.

Sunrise and Sunset - Align Your Subconscious

A Captain can tell a lot about the coming day's weather from the sunrise, and he can prepare for the day ahead to ensure the crew and vessel are best placed to achieve maximum progress towards their destination before any bad weather sets in.

So too with the new dawn each January 1 many of us create New Year's resolutions to change our lives for the coming year. Unfortunately many of us try to act on these resolutions by establishing new habits or a new regime without understanding how best to make sure they stick.

It is often said that habits takes 14 or 28 days to create. If you've ever consciously tried to create a new habit you'll know that you're usually pretty on track for the first few days, but as time goes on it becomes harder and harder to stick to your resolve and often you don't. This happens because your conscious mind that wants the new habit is in conflict with your unconscious mind that doesn't want it.

It is estimated that your brain has 100 billion neurons, electrically excitable cells that process and transmit information by electrical and chemical signalling, and over 100 trillion synapses, or specialised connections with other cells. That's more neural connections than there are grains of sand on the planet. These connections perform all of our conscious or unconscious activities, many automatically via a process called neural coding – that is how the brain's neurons respond to sensory stimuli to produce an outcome in an individual. Everything from breathing to producing a habit.

So the good news is that making a change is as easy as making a new neurological pathway and habits can be created instantly if you have the right tools. All we need to do is recode our neural network to automatically support the habit we want to achieve, without consciously thinking about it. If you drive to work in the same way each day and then someone shows you a shortcut, how long would it take before you start using that shortcut every day? Straight away, right? So too if we employ the right tools and make these connections then we can have instant change.

> *"New habits can be created instantly …*
> *… if you have the right tools."*

But how do you achieve this? How do you reprogram your subconscious?

The human brain operates on four main brainwave levels: Beta, Alpha, Theta and Delta.

Beta brainwaves are the fastest and are an indication of an alert, active, engaged mind. These are the brainwaves you typically experience while you are working and using your conscious brain for non-automatic functioning. You're generally in this state during active and alert periods during the day even up until you head to bed and read for a few minutes.

As we start to get tired our Beta brainwaves slow in to Alpha brainwaves. They are a bit slower and indicate a more relaxed but still engaged state, usually present when you are taking your time, for example when you go for a gentle stroll outside, meditate, or just as you turn off the lights and close your eyes before going to sleep.

After progressing from Beta, our brainwaves slow and pass through Theta to Delta brainwaves which are the slowest and typically occur during sleep, the slowest of which occurs during very deep, restful sleep.

One step up at Theta brainwaves, which are a little faster than Delta but slower that Alpha waves, is where we can harness the power of the subconscious brain. Theta brainwaves are typically associated with daydreaming. If you've ever driven home by automatic pilot and can't actually remember driving home, then you've probably just dipped into Theta state. This is the state in which creativity and new ideas tend to flow from the subconscious to the conscious mind – the brain is open and relaxed and not controlled by the conscious mind or self-talk. Often solutions to complex problems come to people after they've been in this state. And it is here where we can reprogram the subconscious mind.

The best way to access this state is to use audio relaxation techniques. These audio tracks vary in length usually between 10 and 30 minutes and start by relaxing your body and mind. They slowly calm your brainwaves from Beta to Theta rhythm where the suggestive information can plant itself in your subconscious. It's important when you use this technique that you are sitting (or lying) down in a quiet location with dim light, where you won't be disturbed and can truly relax.

Now some people have an issue with the idea of 'reprogramming' – they see it as evil or controlling. But the reality is that the media use more subtle forms of this technique all the time in an effort to get us to buy things that we really don't want or need. I don't know about you, but I'd rather be the one that reprograms my subconscious for the things that I do want. This is why I advocate the use of audio relaxation techniques. In fact I don't believe you can achieve the desired results without their use or regular consultations with a hypnotherapist. There are a huge number of audio tracks available on the market these days that are both convenient and inexpensive, and you can use them again and again and again. The trick is to pick the ones that are going to work for you and are in the format or style that you like, particularly with respect to the background music and more importantly the speaker's voice.

You may find these audio tracks difficult to use at first as your conscious brain does not want to lose control over your body and mind so it can struggle to let go and relax. But if you persist, go with the flow and relax, you will find the process becomes easier with each listen, and you will also move into the Theta state more quickly each time. Remember, you cannot expand your horizons and learn new things until you are prepared to leave your old beliefs behind.

> *"Remember, you cannot discover new oceans unless you have the courage to lose sight of the shore."*

I use these techniques almost every day, and often find I fall asleep during them (which is not the desired result, but it's okay, the information still gets in). But what's really interesting is that I always seem to wake up enough just at the end of the track in time to switch it off. Historically because I have difficulty sleeping (due to an over active brain that's filled with ideas) and because I am so well versed at getting into low Theta waves, I tend to now listen to these tracks after I get into bed, so I can listen to the track and then head straight into delta waves afterwards. It is practical to do this immediately before going to bed because it removes the risk of inadvertently still being in a Theta state at a time when you need to be in an alert Beta state. And I find I get far better quality sleep this way.

What is vital though, is that you never use these techniques while you are engaged in activities that need your full conscious attention, such as driving, operating machinery, even out walking in a park, which might seem a safe enough place to do it, but not if you have to for example, cross a road, negotiate anything or perform any act that requires you to be in a fully alert state.

I've tested many tracks on the market, some are better than others. Head to **www.HalfTheWomanIWas.com** and click on the **VIP** tab for my recommendations for *Relaxation Tracks* that get results.

And best of all, if you have enough courage to use this technique to reprogram your subconscious you will learn the joy of auto pilot, where your subconscious automatically drives you to your goals without any strain or struggle. You'll actually want to get into shape and enjoy the process.

Barnacle Busters – Getting Ship Shape

When a ship is covered with barnacles it produces drag that significantly lowers is speed and efficiency through the water. As the ship's Captain it's important that you get your vessel ship shape and bust any barnacles that are holding you back, clogging up your time and distracting your thoughts and your mind.

Every one of us has a whole list of tasks to complete, so many in fact that we have difficulty remembering them all, and even more difficulty completing the always growing and never ending list. All this stuff that we still have to do is clogging our heads and adding barnacles to our vessel. To get ship shape we need to clear this from our minds as soon as possible.

> *"Increase your efficiency by busting the barnacles that are holding you back."*

First write down all the tasks you have not yet completed, be they small, or incredibly overwhelming; whether they are overdue for completion, or not due for months.

Include any phone calls, letters or emails or "thank you's" still to be communicated. Do you have any broken promises, agreements or lies you need to rectify? Is there anything secret that shouldn't be? Have you got any "once-were-friendships" or soured relationships that are incomplete and need to be properly ended (and I mean in an adult, non-violent manner that will not cause any physical or mental pain to the recipient)?

Is your living space clean and clear? Does your car need a wash or a vacuum and clean out? Is your desk or office a mess?

Look around your home – is there anything you no longer use or wear? Throw or give it away. Do you have things that are broken that haven't yet been fixed? Fix them or throw out anything that can't be fixed.

Have you borrowed something and not returned it yet? Has someone borrowed something from you? Ask for it back as soon as it's appropriate.

Have you balanced your budget lately? Are your personal finances in order? Is your tax overdue? Do you need to make new agreements with any financial institutions? Make sure you organise your financial and legal records. Do you have a will in place and if you have, is it more than three years old or have your circumstances changed? If so then update it - your life is continually evolving and changing and your will should be a reflection of that.

Now think about your primary relationship – are there broken promises, or agreements that you need to make good on? Is there anything that is out of alignment with your ethics, your mind or your body? Write it down now.

Write down anything else you can think of that you should have done, but have never gotten around to doing. Whether it be for work, on the home front, or a volunteer organisation. All those things you promised you'd do, even if the promise was only to yourself.

Now that you have the world's longest list - and rest assured things will continue to pop up, so keep adding them when they do - you can go through and decide whether they a) need to be completed, or b) no longer need to be done.

If they no longer need to be done (e.g. a craft project or repairing an old arm chair), then where practical get rid of anything associated with it, even if it's just the guilt that you have about not doing it. If the task still needs to be done, then prioritise it according to whether it's important, not important, urgent or not urgent.

For the comprehensive *Barnacle Busters Checklist*, prioritisation tips and techniques visit **www.HalfTheWomanIWas.com** and click on the **VIP** tab.

Work through your list each and every day, ticking items off and adding new ones on as they come to you. You will not only bust those barnacles, but you'll be well on the way to achieving your goals.

Navigate By The Stars – Goals and Rewards

Even if a Captain uses auto pilot to drive his vessel, it's vital that he or she learns to navigate by the stars so that from time to time they can look up, check they are on course and make any necessary course corrections. So too you must learn to navigate your brain to ensure your current course is going to lead you to your required destination.

The brain is a complex mechanism, with the conscious and subconscious brain not unlike two siblings. I remember countless trips down to the beach house as a child riding in the back of the car with my older brother, David. When we were getting along we were in unison and it was happy families, everything flowed and the journey was very direct, fun, quiet and reasonably quick.

But when we fought and there was sibling rivalry, each trying to get our parent's attention, it created disharmony, sometimes significant, as we yelled and screamed. Those journeys were incredibly unpleasant and not at all fun, often with detours or stops (sometimes for "toilet stops" which were really an excuse to escape each other for a while). At these times we were warned that if we did not stop our arguing and sniping at each other, the car would be turned around and we would go straight home. Our parents got tired of hearing us whine, "Are we there yet?" because when the journey was tortuous it seemed to go on forever.

As Captain of your ship it's important that you learn how to ensure your brain's conscious and subconscious parts work together in harmony. You need to know what each one requires for this journey, and how to talk with them, in order to produce the best result.

> *"Understanding your subconscious will help you achieve your goals - and rewards - quicker."*

Your conscious brain is your logical brain. It deals with facts and figures and is responsible for your conscious thought, movement and actions. Your conscious brain gets hurt easily by words, and needs lots of support. If you say something negative enough times your conscious brain will start to believe it. Then it will filter into your subconscious and become integrated into your belief system. Talk to your conscious brain positively, Reduce or, preferably, eliminate the negative self-talk. Always say things the way that you want them to be.

Never say you can't do something. People often say they can't afford things. The reality is they probably can afford it, but would probably have to forgo other things, or if it's a large item they may need to go into debt in order to have it. For the most part though, we choose not to have something because it doesn't make financial sense or that some choices are more palatable than others.

Seek clarity within yourself as to why you choose to use certain words and examine the effect they have upon you. Imagine you have some money you've saved and now you need to decide whether you go on holiday to a tropical island, or replace the worn and threadbare carpet in your house. The thought of the island holiday is so alluring; the carpet is just a necessity. "I can't afford both!" you wail to your friends. How does that really make you feel? A failure? Miserable? Hard done by? A victim?

Now rethink the scenario and this time, imagine saying to your friends, "I thought about going on a holiday but have decided to by new carpet for my house, the lounge room will look so much better!" How does that make you feel? Positive and in control? Just by using different words you become someone who is making positive choices to improve your daily life situation. Your thoughts and self-talk can have a profound effect upon your whole life experience. To help change your feelings and self-perceptions, start by changing your words. Rather than saying you can't, say you choose.

Subconsciously the brain can't hear negatives. If you say "I don't want to smoke", all the subconscious brain hears is "I want to smoke" and this then causes the sibling rivalry. The conscious brain wants to stop smoking but the subconscious brain believes you still want to smoke and will do everything in its power to make sure this happens. Instead change it to, "I want to fill my lungs with fresh clean air every moment of every day".

From a goal setting perspective, the single biggest mistake people make when they are writing their goals is to put them in the negative. When you understand how the brain interprets negativity you can understand why these goals never get achieved.

So let's take a moment now to talk about goal setting.

It's time to take your goals from Section 1 and put them into action.

GOALS NEED TO BE S - M - A - R - T

They need to be:

Specific

Measurable

Achievable

Realistic

Time-Oriented

1. Specific

Be definite with the infinite. There's no room for wishy-washy goals in your plan. Make sure they are not only specific, but also simple, concise and clear – no room for misinterpretation or confusion.

Your goals also need to be written in the positive, not the negative. For example, saying you want to lose weight has negative connotations and indicates that you will need to 'find' it again. Instead write that you would like to gain your health and vitality, or that you would like to gain a fit, trim and healthy body.

2. Measurable

This builds on the specific. What's the hard measurable data around your goal? Rather than your goal of "gaining a fit and trim body" put measurable data around it like "I would like to gain a fit, trim and healthy 70kg (154 lbs) body with 22% body fat".

Also, think about where you will be when you achieve your goal – describe it in detail, where are you, what do you see, and how you'll know you have reached it.

For example, "I have a fit, trim and healthy body and I am standing on the scales in my bathroom and the display reads 70kg (154 lbs) and 22% body fat".

3. Achievable

Goals need to be achievable from an ecological perspective. Make sure your goal is safe to you, safe to others and safe to the planet. What comes around goes around – karma will get you. Achieving a goal at the expense of someone or something is unlikely to support you or help you achieve your goal, not in the long term anyhow.

If you are six feet tall and have a goal of 60kg (132 lbs) it's probably not going to be safe to achieve it. Similarly, if you aim to improve your health at the expense of your relationship or job, then that's not going to work either unless you want neither of them – for it will become a self-fulfilling prophecy. You need to ensure your goals are not only supportive of you, but of others too.

When I started my journey, many internet sites advised that for my height I needed to be between 60kg to 65kg (132 lbs to 143 lbs) but I didn't think this was achievable. So I decided on a 10% buffer at 72kg (158 lbs) which seemed more achievable, and within the guidelines for a healthy BMI and other measurements.

4. Realistic

Are your goals realistic and do you think you can achieve them? If you've never achieved your goals in life before then scale them back. If you've always achieved your goals then stretch yourself and make them a little bigger than you normally would.

It can also help to set lots of smaller goals and reset them, rather than just one big goal. You know the old adage. "How do you eat an elephant? – one teaspoon at a time". When I started my journey I couldn't even fathom being less than 100kg (220 lbs) – so my first sub-goal or milestone was to reach 135kg (297 lbs), after which I gradually reset my milestones to lower weights leading down to 100kg (220 lbs) and eventually to my ultimate goal of 72kg (158lbs). Shedding the first 8kg (17lbs) seemed like a much more achievable task than shedding the 72kg (159lbs) that I ultimately did!

Setting smaller achievable goals not only helps with the mental ability to achieve them, it enables you to consistently acknowledge and reward yourself for achieving smaller milestones along the way. This is critical to your motivation and we'll talk a bit more about why this is so important shortly.

5. Time-Oriented

Your goals must be written with a time criteria. To just write " In one year I would like to gain a fit, trim and healthy 70kg (154 lbs) body with 22% body fat" means you'll never get there. Tomorrow, next month and next year never comes. It will be like chasing the pot of gold at the end of the rainbow. To achieve your goals you need to be specific with your time frame.

And use present tense language rather than future tense. For example, "It is 1st January 2019 and I have a fit, trim and healthy body and I am standing on the scales in my bathroom and the display reads 70kg (154 lbs) and 22% body fat and I feel awesome!"

Rewards

Now that you've set your goal we need to discuss the concept of rewards. As Captain it's important that you reward your crew for the hard work they do, and for the goals or milestones they achieve.

Remember when you were a kid you got a reward for behaving well or completing your chores for a whole week without being reminded? My mother had a points system, and for all our chores we received tokens that we could save up and then redeem for items kept we could see high out of reach on the book shelf. Oh how I remember looking up every day at something I wanted, determined to do the right thing and get my tokens in the quickest timeframe possible.

Rewards are not only something that we've all grown up with, they're something that our subconscious is used to receiving. Do the right thing and you'll be rewarded. Use this conditioning to your advantage and set small rewards for small goals.

"If you don't celebrate small, everyday lifestyle changes," says Karen Miller-Kovach, chief scientist at Weight Watchers International, *"there will be times when your long-term weight-loss goal seems so far away that you'll despair or be tempted to give up. Having little stops to celebrate along the way makes that journey more pleasant - and your goal more likely to be achieved"*.

Intrinsically you'll turn to food as a reward, at least initially, rewarding yourself with long lost food friends that you've missed. I know you'll do it because I did it. You'll need to find new ways to reward yourself that don't bring you back into bad habits.

There are lots of choices and not all of them cost money. Here are some to spark your imagination and get your mind spinning with ideas.

- Go and see an old high school friend (you may enjoy their surprised reaction)

- Soak in a long hot bubble bath surrounded by scented candles

- Get a relaxing and pampering massage – good for your soul and it does far more good for your body than you may realise. I get a massage every fortnight as a part of my maintenance routine.

- Indulge in a manicure or pedicure

- Get a completely new haircut or hair style. For one of my sub-goals I got my long hair cut very short. I now prefer short hair over long.

- Get a new look with a makeover with a professional (even if it's just at a department store cosmetics counter)

- Get pierced somewhere new

- Get your teeth whitened

- Buy some new workout clothes

- Buy a new pair of running shoes

- Go shopping and get yourself a new outfit

- Buy a new piece of sexy lingerie

- Get a glamour photo taken

- Buy a special piece of jewellery so every time you wear it you'll remember your success

- Redecorate a room in your house

- Buy a new book you've been wanting to read

- Set aside a whole day to spend reading that new book

- Play some Nintendo Wi or Xbox with a friend – the more active the better

- Go play bingo with your elderly relative or friend (okay that may be a penalty, but you get the idea)

- Take a night off, rent a DVD and snuggle in

- Take a leisurely walk in the park or beautiful gardens

- Go to the museum and learn something new

- Visit a gallery and immerse yourself in some art

- Take a night off and go and see a movie or theatre show

- See a concert you've been wanting to see

- Visit an amusement park and let your inner child out

- Go to the football, rugby or whatever your sporting passion

- Get an adrenalin thrill – jet boat, sky dive or bungee jump, whatever you've always wanted to try but were too afraid to do

- Buy a new (healthy) cook book

- Have your shopping home delivered

- Increase your skills with a cooking class

- Invest in a new healthy kitchen appliance or cooking utensils

- Buy a new CD, play it loud and sing your heart out

- Linger over a cup of tea in a cosy café

- Savour a celebratory glass of wine with dinner

- Phone a distant friend or relative and catch up

- Rent a convertible for a day

- Hire a cleaner or get your ironing done

- Decide on something that you want to buy or do. Whatever the cost break it down into a number of dollars per kilogram you want to lose and set up a savings account. As you shed your kilos your bank balance will grow, and once you reach your goal you'll have the money set aside to enjoy.

The list is as limitless as your imagination.

Along the way I gave myself many rewards including music CDs, new clothes, a new hair style, teeth whitening, aerial gliding training and a hot air balloon ride on a romantic weekend away with my husband.

What have you always wanted to do and would it make a good reward?

Key Learnings

What three qualities do you need to improve as Captain?

1. _______________________________

____

2. _______________________________

____

3. _______________________________

____

What three skills do you need to improve as Captain?

1. _______________________________

____

2. _______________________________

____

3. _______________________________

____

What are the five top barnacles you need to bust?

1. _______________________________________

____

2. _______________________________________

____

3. _______________________________________

____

4. _______________________________________

____

5. _______________________________________

____

What are the five SMART qualities of a goal?

1. _______________________________________

____

2. _______________________________________

____

3. _______________________________________

____

4. _______________________________________

____

5. _______________________________________

____

What are the five top things you are going use to reward yourself?

1. _______________________________________

____

2. _______________________________________

____

3. _______________________________________

____

4. _______________________________________

____

5. _______________________________________

____

Part 3: Reaching Your Destination

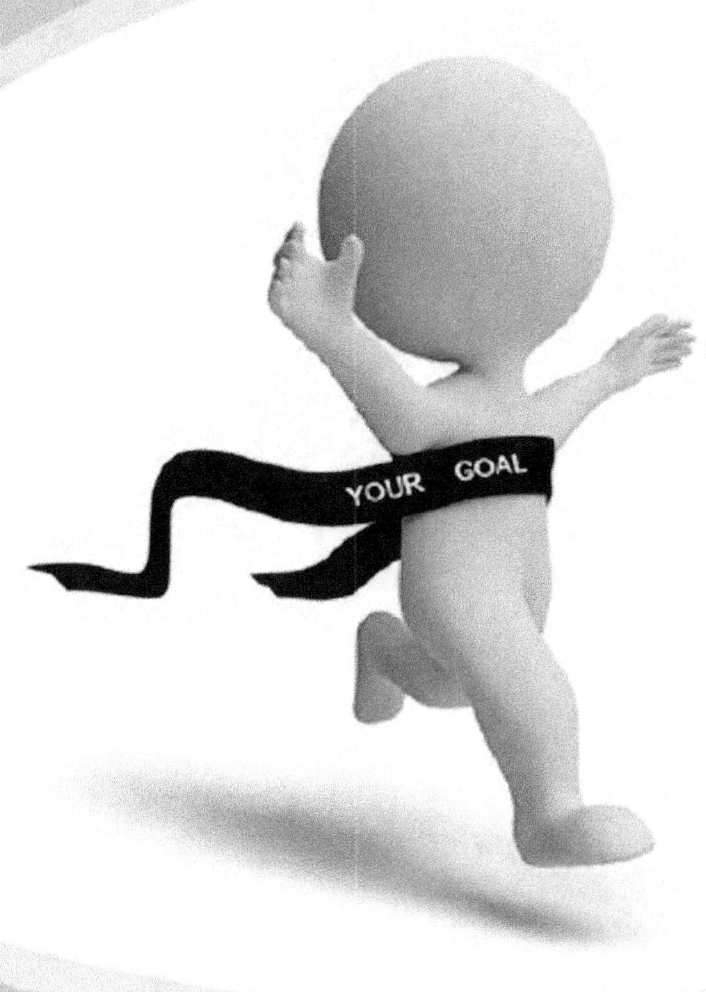

9. Putting It All Together

Now that you've completed your Itinerary in *Get Your Mind Right*, *Get Your Body Right* and *Get Your Spirit Right* you're ready to put everything together and reach for your destination.

Take a minute to think about all that you've learned so far… How much of what you were doing wasn't supporting your dream? How many things were you doing to yourself that were actually causing you damage and taking you further away from your goals?

How much more do you know now and how much more confident are you that you can make changes for the better and improve your health and vitality?

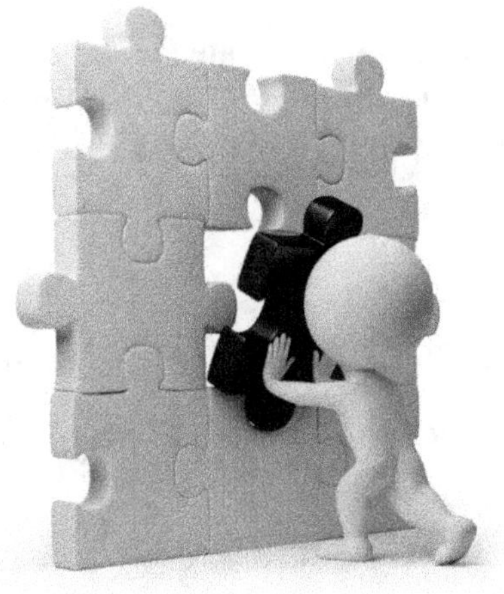

Remember to start simply with small changes – don't try and do everything all at once or you'll blow yourself, your friends and your family all out of the water. Make a commitment to stick to your itinerary for at least the first month. Review your task lists daily and make sure you measure your progress weekly.

Once you start to see your progress you'll get on a roll and the next month won't be so hard. Have you ever noticed that when you wake up and the first few morning tasks flow, that the rest of the day tends to be a good day, but when you have a bad morning things seem to go from bad to worse? A lot of this is mind over matter – your perception colours reality to an extent.

In weight loss, when you are successful you tend to be doing the right things that produce the right results and when you actually start seeing the results it puts you on a high and you become more optimistic, making it much easier to keep doing the right things. As you a accomplish more and more, you'll believe in yourself and will begin to believe your goal is attainable. You'll have heaps more energy and life will become less of a struggle. Yes, everything will then flow, and be easy breezy lemon squeezy. After a while your hunger for success will engulf you and you'll be unstoppable.

It vital to stay motivated on this journey – do it for your spouse, do it for your kids, do it to fit into that little black dress you've had your eye on. But most of all, do it for yourself. You deserve to be all that you can be.

> *"Do it for any reason that works, but most of all do it for yourself - you deserve to be all that you can be."*

Having goals will give you a sense of purpose and make the week easier – no more Monday-itis (take that Bob Geldof!). Once you're in motion and have developed momentum you'll want to keep going. And once others start seeing the results and your friends gasp, "Wow, you look great!" you'll be feeling on top of the world and you'll actually encourage others to start achieving their goals – if you can do it so can they. You'll become a role model for others.

As you keep going on your journey keep referring back to the required sections of this book – you'll keep learning and, over time, all this knowledge will become second nature.

Once again I guarantee the road ahead won't always be easy. I guarantee at times the challenges ahead may even be quite painful. I guarantee along the way you will have doubts and you may even want to give up.

Write your goals down clearly and review them daily. Discard negative language and behaviour. Create personal challenges, use affirmations, positive language, positive motivation, and reinforcement to support achieving your goals.

Remember to ignore the things that are unimportant – don't get distracted by things that will take your focus from your goal and deplete your energy reserves. I virtually never watch the news reports or read a newspaper – it's all sensationalism anyway and if I really need to know something someone will tell me. Plus it's a great conversation starter to have someone give you their version of events. Ignore the unimportant – you need all your energy for you.

Understand what makes you bored and make sure you have a list of things to do if you are. Boredom is an energy zapper and motivation destroyer. I'm far too busy to be bored these days – I work my long task list and keep adding to it every day. Someone once said, "God put me on this earth to accomplish a certain number of things, and right now I'm so far behind I'll never die". Keep yourself busy and switch tasks if you find your current one hard to complete. Just a change of pace can help clear your mind, allowing you to return to the original task with a fresh approach.

Regularly measure your progress and track your results. If you find your spirits flagging then grab the record of your breakthroughs and review it. You'll be so impressed with all you've achieved your spirit will start to soar again. Also reading inspirational books and the success stories of others can be a great mood enhancer and you may even pick up a few tips along the way. Don't forget to reward your achievements; you will create an automatic motivator to get to your next goal.

Keep in mind that for every action there is an equal and opposite reaction. If you're down, getting into motion will raise your spirits, and none more so than a little exercise. Get active and get your share of endorphins – nature's happiness drug. Remember to spend a little time outside each day communing with nature and getting valuable sunshine. If you're still finding it hard then turn your favourite song on for an instant mood changer.

Clean your personal space and allow for the flow of creativity and energy. An uncluttered space is an uncluttered mind. Live in integrity. Ensure you keep all of the promises or agreements you've made - keep your commitments or make new ones. Focus on one thing at a time if you're feeling overwhelmed – you'll soon get through that list - but remember to make sure it's quality and not quantity.

Remember laughter makes the world go around so read or watch comedies or just have some fun with your friends. It's a great stress reliever and will keep your spirits up. And avoid people who suck your energy and make you feel down – negative people and those who say you can't are simply playing power games by putting you down in order to bolster themselves up. They will drain your energy quicker than you can replenish it. Instead look for positive people – they're much more fun and energising to be around.

Learn to say "no" to things that don't support you. Many times we continually try to please everyone around us, saying yes and making all manner of promises we don't really want to make. Start being more selective and say no from time to time in a polite nice manner – odds on you'll find it quite liberating.

Don't aim for perfection. Accept that things can be difficult and sometimes you won't succeed. Don't dwell on your feeling of failure or dissatisfaction. Fallen off the horse? Get back in the saddle, partner!

> *"Don't seek perfection ~*
> *just aim to improve a little each day."*

Along your journey there'll be many changes, one of which is your body will start to shrink and it will change shape. I went from a size 30 to a size 10. Several months after I started losing weight I found all my clothes were far too big and baggy and I looked fatter than I really was. So I went to a retail clothing store bought a couple of new pairs of trousers and several new shirts. I spent a fair amount of money only to find about eight weeks later they were too big for me too!

During the weight loss phase it was often difficult and at times frustrating to know what size to buy, not to mention the wasted cost when I out-shrank them! I found it a much better solution was to go to a charity recycled clothing store. Not only can you find good quality clothing, you'll sometimes pick up designer brands at a fraction of the price. You do need to pick through the clothing on offer, but you'll also get a chance to try on colours and shapes that you would never have looked at previously and you can end up creating a whole new look for yourself.

Set aside a few hours to try on clothes and check the quality of each garment to ensure they're not faulty or stained. Don't forget to donate your "fat" clothes back to the store – you won't need them any longer and they may give you a discount on future purchases. Once you have your haul, wash them thoroughly and include some disinfectant liquid and eucalyptus oil in the wash to freshen them up.

If you are having issues with loose baggy skin, it takes time to shrink (often a year or two and it's another reason not to attempt to lose weight too quickly), so you need to practice patience. In the meantime start doing some resistance training to tone up, and use massage creams or oils daily that are designed to repair scar and post pregnancy stretch marks - it will help. Compression garments can also assist in supporting the skin during the shrinking process. I regularly wore compression running garments underneath my clothes to help lift everything and stop the wobble. On occasion I still wear them.

If after a significant period of time you are still having excess skin issues then you may need to consult a plastic surgeon. Cosmetic surgery is a major step, it should not be entered into lightly but used as a last resort where everything else has been tried first. A good surgeon will only suggest a procedure if it is going to produce a significant benefit. Two years after I achieved my goal weight I still had huge folds of skin on my stomach, giving me a tummy that I would otherwise not have had. So I decided to have abdominoplasty to remove the excess skin, but it was a serious decision and an expensive procedure, much of it not being covered by health funds or Medicare. I am thrilled with the result and my hip to hip scar has faded nicely over the years.

10. The Secret to Success – Final Words

I hate to break your bubble of illusion but the greatest secret is that there is no quick fix! Success takes continuous action, daily commitment, determination and courage – all often disguised as hard work. Andrew Carnegie said, *"Anything in life worth having is worth working for!"*

The reason 99% of people don't succeed is lack of knowledge and lack of desire – so they just quit. You are now armed with all the knowledge you need to succeed, so step up and be the 1% that achieves your dreams, your desires and your goals.

It's now time to stop reading and get into action! Remember you don't need to go on this journey alone. There are lots of family and friends who will support you – if you only ask. And there's a whole website I've designed with you in mind, specifically to hold your hand on this journey. So get surfing and go to **www.HalfTheWomanIWas.com** Check out what's on offer and decide what's going to work for you and help you get you to your goals sooner.

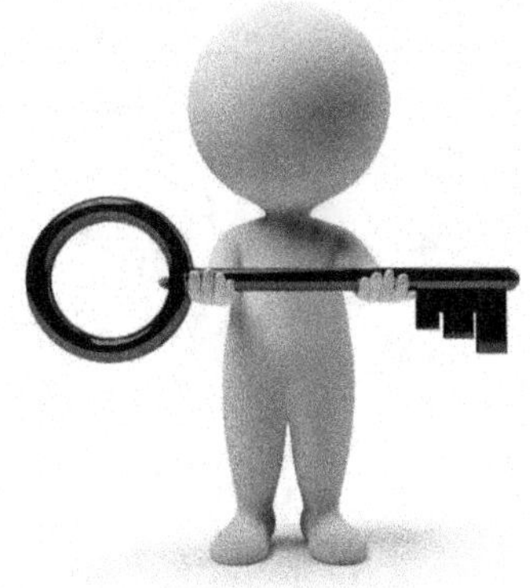

Also on my website is a comprehensive a *Resources Directory*. I have hand-picked and fully endorse all the products and services listed. Most of them are ones I have personally used on my journey. I've even managed to twist some arms and many of them have been good enough to offer you a discount.

If, after all that, you're still having significant trials and tribulations, or are really stuck, then contact me through my website and I or one of my team will help get you through. And when you do get to your goal don't forget to contact me and let me know your success stories – I want to celebrate your success too!

If you haven't started already, then isn't it time to get into action now? But before we say "Bon Voyage" there's one last thing I'd like to leave you with - a famous poem that was written many years ago by an unknown author. This poem is very special to me and really sums up what we all need to do when following our dreams.

DON'T QUIT

When things go wrong, as they sometimes will,

When the road you're trudging seems all uphill,

When the funds are low and the debts are high,

And you want to smile, but you have to sigh,

When care is pressing you down a bit,

Rest, if you must, but don't you quit.

Life is queer with its twists and turns,

As every one of us sometimes learns,

And many a failure turns about,

When he might have won had he stuck it out;

Don't give up though the pace seems slow –

You may succeed with another blow.

Often the goal is nearer than,

It seems to a faint and faltering man,

Often the struggler has given up,

When he might have captured the victor's cup,

And he learned too late when the night slipped down,

How close he was to the golden crown.

Success is failure turned inside out –

The silver tint of the clouds of doubt,

And you never can tell how close you are,

It may be near when it seems so far,

So stick to the fight when you're hardest hit

It's when things seem worst that you must not quit.

- Author unknown

About The Author

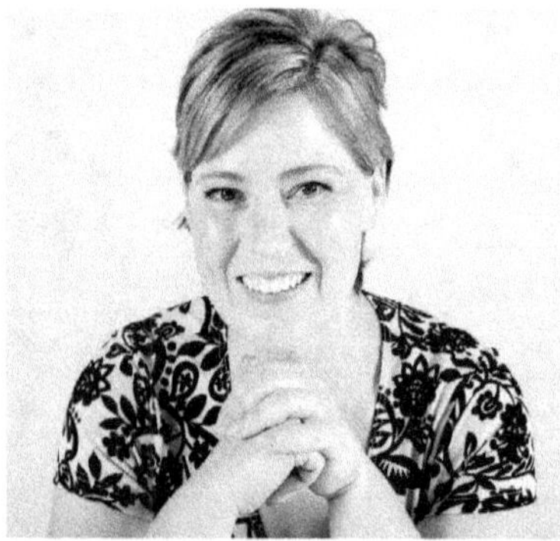

Sigrid de Castella grew up an obese child in a family of famous athletes. The ridicule and shame she experienced as a young child followed her into her 20s and 30s until she finally found the courage to change. Her search for the truth led her to realise the trauma of the sexual abuse she'd experienced as a child - at the hands of a family acquaintance - was not the only thing keeping her fat.

Armed with a newfound knowledge she began to tear down the protective wall she'd built around herself, brick by brick and set about changing her weight and her life. The result is a most remarkable transformation. Sigrid lost over 70kg (150 pounds) - more than half her body weight - without surgery and without 'dieting'.

In the 20 month journey Sigrid not only discovered the secret to life-long health and vitality, she discovered how to regain her life and re-build it from the ground up to achieve a new sense of freedom, love and happiness.

With a personal knowledge of how painful it is to be judged by your looks and your weight rather than your abilities, Sigrid is determined to share her secrets with others, so they too can achieve their full potential. It is her desire to inspire others to reach their dreams that drives Sigrid to write, speak and mentor.

Apart from being a recognised authority in the field of health and weight loss, Sigrid is also a highly successful business woman, entrepreneur and an accomplished photographer who has been capturing the world around her for more than 20 years. Her images can be seen at www. worldimageart.com

Sigrid lives in Melbourne, Australia with her husband, Antony, and their two dogs, Kimba and Willow.

Become a VIP
(Very Important Passenger)
Visit the website and click on the VIP tab.
Password: success

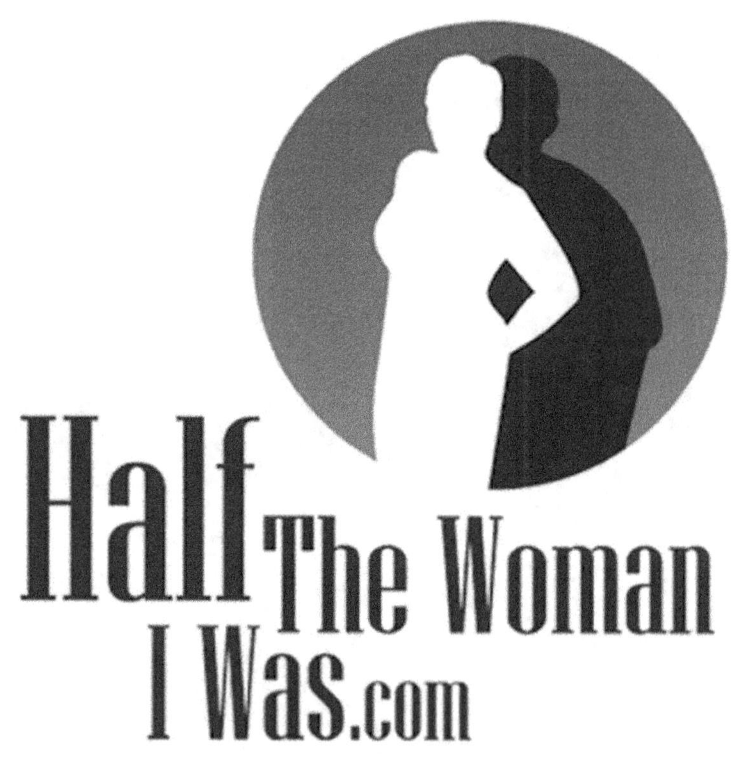

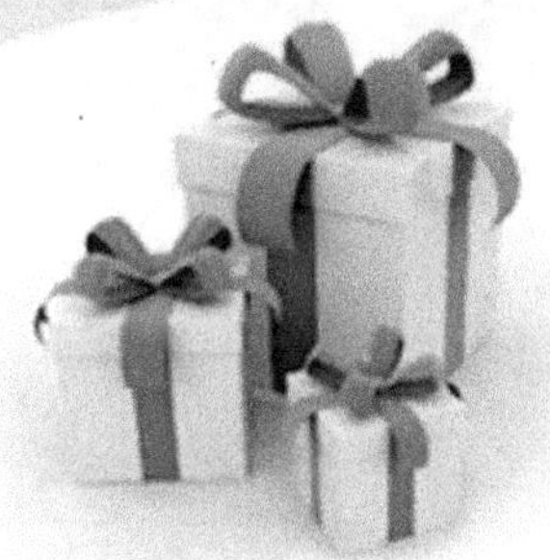

Your Free VIP Gifts
Worth over $3,000.00!

VIP Bonus #1
Review of Body Fat Scales   *$79 value*

VIP Bonus #2
Review of Diet Diaries   *$79 value*

VIP Bonus #3
Lifestyle Profile and free report   *$357 value*

VIP Bonus #4
Unlimited access to HTWIW Complete Body Calculator   *$579 value*

VIP Bonus #5
Medical Risk Profile and free report   *$357 value*

VIP Bonus #6
HTWIW Simple Eating Plan   *$149 value*

VIP Bonus #7
HTWIW Resistance Training Program   *$197 value*

VIP Bonus #8
HTWIW Stretching Guide   *$197 value*

VIP Bonus #9
Unlimited Access to HTWIW Stress Test and free Report   *$579 value*

VIP Bonus #10
HTWIW Barnacle Busters Checklist   *$249 value*

VIP Bonus #11
HTWIW Resources Directory, Discounts and Offers   *Unlimited value*

VIP Bonus #12
A year of HTWIW Motivational Images   *$197 value*